The Field Analyzer Primer:
Effective Perimetry

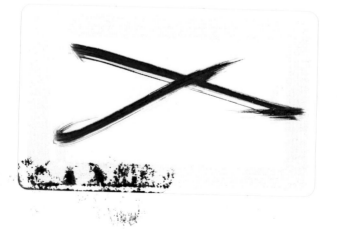

The Field Analyzer Primer: Effective Perimetry

FOURTH EDITION

Anders Heijl, MD PhD
Professor and Chairman
Dept. of Ophthalmology
Lund University
Skåne University Hospital
Malmö, Sweden

Vincent Michael Patella, OD
Vice President, Professional Affairs
Carl Zeiss Meditec, Inc.
Dublin, California

Boel Bengtsson, PhD
Associate Professor
Dept. of Ophthalmology
Lund University
Skåne University Hospital
Malmö, Sweden

Carl Zeiss Meditec, Inc.
5160 Hacienda Drive
Dublin, California 94568, USA
+1 925.557.4100
Toll-Free 877.486.7473

Carl Zeiss Meditec AG
Goeschwitzer Strasse 51-52
D-07745 Jena, Germany
Phone: +49.3641.220.0

Cover design: Johan Heijl
Text design and composition: Seventeenth Street Studios
Illustrations and infographics: Johan Heijl
Photos: Johan Heijl
Index: Janet Perlman

Contents

Foreword

THIS NEW EDITION OF *The Field Analyzer Primer* is timely. Since the previous edition, there have been improvements in perimetric software, but more importantly we now have a better understanding of the meaning of certain results. Test results, for example, no longer should be viewed as either reliable or unreliable, but as falling on a continuum from highly reliable to marginally informative, sometimes containing useful information even when indicators of reliability are not optimal. We now understand that False Positive responses—when the patient presses the response button even when no stimulus has been seen—are more destructive to interpretation than formerly believed, that the gaze tracker probably provides more accurate measures of patient fixation stability than does the blind spot method, and that False Negative responses are to be expected in distinctly abnormal fields, even when patients have been highly attentive to the test.

In a similar way, progression is no longer viewed as simply being present or absent, but careful evaluation will consider the rate of change, as well as the degree of certainty that change really has occurred. Both diagnosis and management can now be better than ever before when a modern automated perimeter is used in an astute manner by a well-informed practitioner.

The first two editions of this primer—published more than 20 years ago—concentrated on perimetric technology, however complex. The third edition, written in 2002, looked more at how to simplify and standardize the clinical process. This new edition seeks to emphasize the insights of the last decade, including not only those just mentioned, but also the importance of human interaction during testing and the importance of quantifying change as a rate rather than simply as an event when a change from baseline can be recognized.

The reader has the good fortune that this primer has been written by the people who have been largely responsible for the development and continual improvement of the Humphrey perimeter. You should not pass up the opportunity to learn from them by reading this work and using it for reference from time to time. In the modern world, most of us operate new computerized devices by intuition, without ever reading the instruction manual. However, when using a modern perimeter, it often is important to understand the workings of the instrument, as well as the nature of visual defects from disease (and artifacts). This primer was written to address these essentials, but experience and further study also will help the reader achieve and maintain up-to-date expertise.

I remember when testing of visual fields was performed manually, most typically by the physician himself, at a tangent screen, with an effort by some to carefully calibrate the room illumination level and to record results quantitatively, in terms of the size of the round white bead contrasting with the black background. Then came manual perimeters designed by people like Aulhorn with Harms in Tübingen and Goldmann in Bern, with carefully calibrated illumination of the stimulus and background. John Lynn may have been the first to attempt to have the test conducted automatically using emerging technology that was primitive by today's standards. Quite a number of automated perimeters were developed, with increasing sophistication. In the decades since, we have seen improved test accuracy, shortened test times, and the addition of statistical analyses to help both with diagnosis and with monitoring for change. Lost in that process is the art of performing the test, and as importantly the practitioner's thoughtful involvement as the test is being conducted. It need not be so with automated perimetry if the perimetrist and practitioner each undertake their tasks insightfully.

For the conduct of the test, Chapter 2 is particularly important, because it explains how the perimetrist can improve test results, even when using a highly automated instrument. The perimetrist should not simply stand by and watch the machine conduct the test, but should perform the test using the instrument. With that mind-set, the perimetrist ensures that the patient understands what the test is going to be like, is positioned correctly, has the proper lens correction in place, is comfortable and alert, is maintaining fixation centrally, and so on. A brief word of encouragement from time to time keeps the patient alert and attentive to the task. The quality of the examination is highly dependent on the perimetrist, and experienced expert perimetrists routinely recognize when adjustments are needed, or when the patient needs a brief pause for rest.

The practitioner, for his part, should have undergone perimetric testing at least once to appreciate the nature of the task performed by the patient, and to understand the sources of artifacts, both to instruct the perimetrist and to recognize artifacts mixed within the diagnostically useful information on the printed report, which includes increasingly helpful statistical analyses.

Please reward yourself and your patients by absorbing the contents of this primer, growing further in your expertise with experience, and by staying current with even newer information as it becomes available.

Douglas R. Anderson, MD, FARVO
Professor Emeritus, Bascom Palmer Eye Institute
University of Miami Miller School of Medicine
Miami, Florida, USA
October 2012

Preface

AUTOMATED PERIMETRY WAS JUST gaining acceptance 25 years ago when the first edition of this primer was published. That text emphasized technical and psychophysical topics and contemplated a wide spectrum of possible testing options. Today, clinical perimetry has become much more standardized, and this new edition concentrates on the specific procedures that over the years have been incorporated into the worldwide standard of care.

Today, we believe that the most immediate opportunities for improving automated perimetry lie in the areas of perimetrist training and patient instruction and supervision. These topics are so important that we have devoted a whole new chapter to discussing them. If you read only one chapter in this book, we hope it will be Chapter 2, "Effective Perimetry."

Chapters 6 and 8 also are new, and reflect the growing importance of measuring progression—and especially perimetric progression—in glaucoma management. These chapters reflect our own interpretation of what we believe to be the most significant advances in glaucoma management philosophy in the last 15 years. We provide a number of citations addressing this area, and encourage the reader to consider the topic more broadly.

The last 10 years have seen the rapid refinement and adoption of automated imaging techniques that today quite effectively complement the information provided by automated perimetry. Thus, it is fitting that we have added a new section—Chapter 9—that considers the relationship between structural and functional measurements in glaucoma management.

This new edition, *Effective Perimetry,* continues to limit itself to clinical perimetry as it is presently practiced worldwide. We have adopted this narrow focus in order to provide students, residents, and busy practitioners with clear and succinct suggestions for effective use of perimetry in everyday patient care. However, readers should also understand that the authors see clinical perimetry as a continuously evolving discipline and an area of diagnostics that once again is attracting international scientific attention. In partial recognition of these facts, we have expanded this edition's list of references in order to encourage readers who wish also to delve into scientific topics not addressed in this primer.

On a personal note, this fourth edition celebrates 30 years of collaboration between its three coauthors in the development of clinical perimetry. We wish to recognize and thank those who have helped us along the way—a list too long to be recorded here. We especially wish to recognize the author of the Foreword to this edition, Professor Douglas R. Anderson. Professor Anderson has been our collaborator, mentor, and friend for almost all of those 30 years. We also wish to recognize Professor Stephen M. Drance, who has helped us immeasurably from the very beginning. To both, we send our thanks and our best wishes.

Anders Heijl, MD, PhD
Vincent Michael Patella, OD
Boel Bengtsson, PhD
October 2012

Introduction: How to Use this Primer

THIS BOOK IS INTENDED to serve as an introduction to clinical automated perimetry and particularly visual field testing using the Humphrey perimeter. It has been written as a concise introduction and reference that may be used by busy practitioners and in training programs.

Because of its purpose, this primer does not follow the outline of most textbooks. For example, the bare essentials of modern practical perimetry are covered in a very condensed form in Chapter 1.

Those who only have time for absolutely basic information may choose just to read Chapter 1 and to refer to the other chapters as the need may arise. Others may choose to read the book in its entirety—a task that we hope will not be very time-consuming.

We do, however, strongly recommend that you also read Chapter 2, "Effective Perimetry." This chapter addresses what we believe to be the single most fertile area for improving clinical perimetry—the management and training of patients and technical staff.

1

The Essentials of Perimetry

THIS CHAPTER PROVIDES A quick outline of essential perimetric facts. The topics presented here are treated more fully in later chapters.

What is Automated Static Perimetry?

Automated threshold static perimetry quantifies the sensitivity of a patient's peripheral vision using efficient and standardized testing algorithms. While perimeters usually are also capable of performing suprathreshold testing—in which the only goal is to confirm that visual function is not below the normal range—the main function of these devices is precise quantification.

When Is Perimetry Called For?

Perimetry is essential in glaucoma management. It also is frequently useful in diagnosing and managing neurological diseases, and it has a role in the diagnosis and management of some retinal diseases. Perimetry also is used to certify visual function, such as quantifying a patient's level of visual disability or ability to drive.

GLAUCOMA

Perimetry is fundamental in glaucoma diagnosis and management. Perimetric test results that reproducibly demonstrate visual field loss remain the most conclusive contributor to glaucoma diagnosis. Even now, in the second decade of the 21st century, the most precise method for quantifying glaucomatous progression remains repeated visual field testing. Imaging-based measurements of the optic disc, retinal nerve fiber layer, and ganglion cells are nevertheless increasingly important, and provide information that clearly is complementary to perimetry.

NEUROLOGICAL DISEASE

When managing neurological disease, field testing is not as crucial a technique as it is in glaucoma management; neuroimaging often can replace perimetry. Nevertheless, visual field testing may sometimes provide an inexpensive and noninvasive alternative to neuroimaging and a way of documenting changes in visual function.

RETINAL DISEASE

Visual field testing has a role in the diagnosis and management of some retinal diseases, but direct observation and imaging of the fundus usually are of greater value. Perimetry then becomes one of many ancillary tests. Peripheral visual field testing may play a somewhat larger role in retinal disease than it does in glaucoma or neurological disease.

What Are We Looking for?

GLAUCOMATOUS VISUAL FIELD LOSS

Glaucomatous visual field loss frequently occurs first in the so-called Bjerrum areas which follow an arcuate course from the blind spot, coursing above and below the macula, and ending at the temporal raphe. Early glaucomatous field defects most often take the form of localized relative scotomas, i.e., small areas of decreased sensitivity. Defects in the nasal field are particularly common, and sensitivity differences across the nasal horizontal meridian often are diagnostically useful (Fig 7-4).

Perimetric testing of glaucoma patients is seldom done in the area outside the central 30° field. Only a small percentage of glaucomatous defects occur in the peripheral field alone, and testing the central 25°–30° field is preferred in glaucoma management today.

Considerable test-retest variability is a hallmark of areas of the visual field affected by glaucomatous visual field loss; variable sensitivity reductions occurring in the same area, but not always at the same test point locations, commonly precede clear-cut glaucomatous field defects (Fig 5-2). Although a reduction in overall visual field sensitivity frequently is seen in combination with localized glaucomatous loss, purely homogeneous reductions are more commonly associated with cataract or drug-induced miosis—and thus usually are too nonspecific to be relied upon in glaucoma diagnosis (Fig 7-8).

NEUROLOGICAL VISUAL FIELD LOSS

Most neurological field defects are hemianopic, that is, they tend to affect either the right half of the visual field or the left and to respect the vertical meridian. As with glaucoma, the great majority of defects start in the central 30° of the visual field, and thus central visual field testing is preferred here as well (Chapter 10).

RETINAL VISUAL FIELD LOSS

Visual field testing sometimes is used to test for a variety of field defects caused by retinal disease. Such defects are often deep, with steep borders (Fig 11-2), and may occur in any part of the visual field.

COEXISTING DISEASE

Because glaucoma patients frequently also develop retinal and neurological disease, it is important to be able to recognize the development of retinal and neurological field defects, even if those diseases are not primarily managed using perimetry.

Selecting a Test

Threshold testing is always a good choice, and in ophthalmic clinical settings it is almost always to be preferred over suprathreshold screening tests. Threshold testing can detect the earliest visual field changes and is also the standard of care for following patients who have established field loss.

We recommend use of the 24-2 test pattern and the Swedish Interactive Thresholding Algorithm (SITA) Standard thresholding strategy for most patients, and that you depart from these only when necessary. In any case, we recommend that each clinician—and preferably each clinic—standardize on a preferred test pattern and testing strategy. Such standardization facilitates test-to-test comparability. The 24-2 pattern tests 54 locations and is identical to the 30-2 pattern except that most of the outermost ring of points has been removed (Fig 4-1).

The SITA Standard strategy offers high accuracy and relatively short test times of 3 to 7 minutes per eye. SITA Fast is a very fast threshold test that usually takes 2 to 5 minutes per eye and offers slightly less, but still high, accuracy, especially in experienced patients.[29, 30, 32–37] Contrary to popular belief, SITA Fast is not a simpler test for the patient than SITA Standard. In the interest of optimal efficiency and speed, SITA Fast was designed to present stimuli that are only subtly visible, therefore requiring finer discrimination on the part of the patient than does SITA Standard. SITA Fast is a very effective test in experienced patients and in younger patients, however.

PERIMETRIC FOLLOW-UP

It is usually best to follow a patient over time using the same test that was used for diagnosis. If a patient is consistently examined with the same test strategy and test pattern, then tests can be more easily compared using standardized progression analyses (Chapter 6).

PERIPHERAL FIELD TESTING

While the Humphrey Field Analyzer (HFA) has complete capabilities for testing in the peripheral field, automated testing peripheral to 30° from fixation is rarely performed for diagnostic purposes. Peripheral suprathreshold testing is mostly used to determine visual function in drivers and to establish the level of visual disability for insurance purposes. Note that the goal in such certification testing is quite different from the usual goals when diagnosing and managing disease, in that the former usually is done in order to assess significant loss, while the latter seeks to detect and quantify subtle defects and small amounts of change over time.

OTHER TESTS

In advanced glaucoma, it may be helpful to concentrate testing in the remaining central field by shifting to the 10-2 pattern (Fig 4-4A–B), or to change to a larger size V stimulus (Fig 4-4C–D). The HFA II offers a selection of specific, functional tests that are sometimes needed for legal purposes. These tests and their uses may differ from country to country.

Interpreting the Results

One of the advantages of Humphrey perimetry is that there is a whole package of STATPAC analyses that are automatically applied to the results of standard Humphrey threshold tests. STATPAC can help to identify visual fields that fall outside the normal range, to identify patients whose vision continues to deteriorate, and to determine the rate of disease progression. Needless to say, analysis of test results only makes sense if those results have been accurately associated with the correct patient, and software systems are now available that reduce patient identification errors by linking the HFA to centralized databases (Fig 13-2). The following description identifies important STATPAC features. Further suggestions for interpreting these results are found in Chapters 5 and 6.

Useful STATPAC Analyses (Fig 1-1)

TOTAL DEVIATION MAPS

Decibel deviations from age-corrected normal sensitivities are shown in the Total Deviation numerical plot. More importantly, the associated Total Deviation probability map highlights deviations that fall outside the statistical range of normal sensitivity.

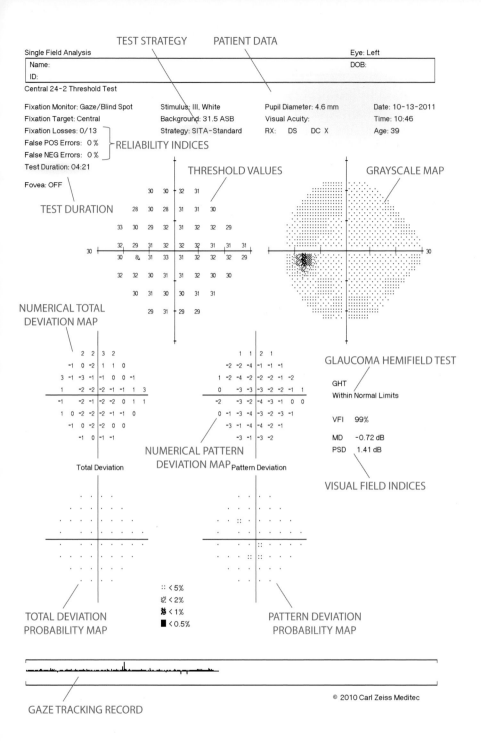

Figure 1-1

Sample STATPAC Single Field Analysis (SFA) from an eye with a normal visual field.

PATTERN DEVIATION MAPS

The Pattern Deviation maps highlight localized loss after first correcting for any overall change in the height of the hill of vision, such as that caused by cataract. Decibel deviations from expected values are shown in the upper numeric plot, while the statistical significance of those deviations is shown in the accompanying probability plot. The Pattern Deviation probability plot may be the single most useful STATPAC analysis when glaucoma is suspected.

NUMERICAL THRESHOLD SENSITIVITIES

This presentation simply shows the measured decibel sensitivity at each tested point, and is the basic information upon which all the other analyses and printouts are based (Fig 3-3).

GRAYSCALE PRINTOUTS

The grayscale is an intuitive way of presenting raw decibel sensitivity, with dark areas indicating reduced sensitivity. However, because the data are not compared to normal ranges, significant loss may be unrecognizable in this presentation. Perhaps the most important use of this presentation is in depicting artifactual loss (Chapter 12) and profound visual field defects.

THE GLAUCOMA HEMIFIELD TEST (GHT)

This is an expert system for analyzing threshold test results. It has been reported to detect glaucomatous visual field loss with both high sensitivity and high specificity and expresses its analysis in plain language.[47, 64] This may be the single best place to look for practitioners who are not highly experienced at visual field analysis, when judging whether a test result is normal or pathological in a glaucoma patient or suspect. The GHT was not designed to be sensitive to neurological or retinal field loss.

VISUAL FIELD INDICES (MD, VFI, AND PSD)

Mean Deviation (MD) is a weighted average of the values presented in the Total Deviation numerical plot, with 0 indicating no deviation from normal and large negative values being associated with advanced field loss. Visual Field Index (VFI) is an enhancement of MD that is designed to be less affected by cataract and more sensitive to changes near the center of the field, in order to better correlate with ganglion cell loss. Normal vision is associated with VFI values near 100%, while perimetric blindness produces VFI values approaching 0%. Pattern Standard Deviation (PSD) summarizes localized loss in a single index, while ignoring generalized depression. PSD is low for normal fields, for uniformly depressed fields and for blind fields, and is highest in moderate to advanced localized loss.

These indices usually are less helpful for diagnosis than the probability maps and the GHT. However, VFI and MD are very helpful for staging and following patients over time; the newer VFI index being, in our view, preferable. Levels of statistical significance compared to normal are shown next to MD and PSD values that fall outside the normal range. VFI does not show normative significance limits, because it was developed primarily as a staging and progression metric.

Progressive Visual Field Change

Glaucoma management relies heavily on the quantification of visual field change over time. The Guided Progression Analysis (GPA) discussed in Chapters 6 and 8 has been designed to help practitioners identify and quantify visual field progression. GPA has two types of analyses: Glaucoma Change Probability Maps and the VFI trend analysis. These two analyses are presented together in standardized GPA reports. Our favorite is the GPA Summary Report (Fig 1-2).

Glaucoma Change Probability Maps are designed to identify progression events. They show areas of the tested field that have changed by more than the range of testing variability typically found in most glaucoma patients. Reproducible statistically significant changes may be associated with glaucomatous progression.

Regression analysis of summary parameters such as VFI or MD, on the other hand, are trend analyses that help differentiate between patients progressing at dangerously rapid rates versus patients who may be progressing so slowly as to not require more aggressive intervention.

During the last few years a paradigm shift has occurred in glaucoma management. While perimetric follow-up used to focus primarily on whether or not visual field progression had occurred, we now are also interested in determining the patient's rate of progression. The reason for this shift is that long-term studies have shown that most treated glaucoma patients do progress, and that progression usually will be evident if perimetric testing has been performed at reasonable test intervals. Today, we try to differentiate between patients who are progressing rapidly and dangerously—and who need increasingly aggressive therapy—versus patients who are progressing so slowly that a change in therapy is neither necessary nor appropriate.

Overview printouts (Fig 5-8) can facilitate qualitative review of many tests over time.

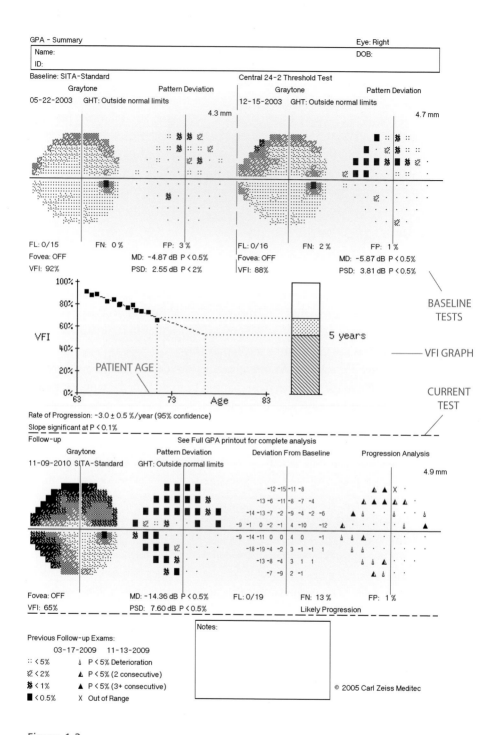

Figure 1-2

Guided Progression Analysis (GPA) Summary Report analysis from an eye with progressive glaucomatous visual field loss.

Common Interpretation Pitfalls

Several typical patterns of artifactual test results are worth recognizing. These include fields from eyes with partial ptosis or prominent eyebrows, fields in which the correction lens or lens holder has blocked the patient's peripheral vision and produced a false field defect, fields from patients who anxiously pressed the response button even when no stimulus was seen ("trigger-happy" fields), and so-called cloverleaf fields that are characteristic of patients who ceased paying attention early in the test. Learning effects occur in patients who are new to perimetry, but are typically small. A minority of patients may produce results characterized by concentric contraction or peripheral reduction of sensitivity. Such artifactual contractions are the exception and are considerably less common in 24-2 fields than in 30-2 fields. These and other features of the test results are discussed more fully in Chapter 12.

2

Effective Perimetry

MANY YEARS OF THOUGHT and development have gone into making automated perimetry as simple and effective as possible. While some have suggested that perimetry is difficult for both the patient and the professional, we do not at all agree. There are clear attitudes and processes that can minimize such difficulties. In this chapter we will present suggestions that may help make perimetry simpler and more effective in your clinic.

Attitudes That Can Promote Success

Perimetry is automated, but patients are not. Most patients can and will produce reliable results if they just understand why perimetry is being performed, what to expect, and what they need to do.[1] The key to positive patient performance lies in staff behavior, attitudes, and skill. Instilling positive attitudes in patients and staff probably is the most important step you can take to make perimetry effective and trouble free in your practice.

STAFF MEMBERS WILL HAVE A POSITIVE ATTITUDE TOWARD PERIMETRY

- If they understand the role of perimetry in therapeutic decision making.
- If their doctors have taken a personal interest in their perimetry training and have shown positive expectations about the process.
- If they have personally taken perimetry tests and are able to communicate their experiences to patients.
- If they understand the importance of patient emotional and physical comfort.
- If they are confident in their perimetric skills.

- If they understand the goals of visual field testing and its importance in their care.
- If they realize that the instrument is programmed to dim the stimulus until they no longer can see it, that they probably will see the light less than half the time, and that when they do see the light it probably will be quite dim.
- If they are comfortably positioned at the perimeter and reassuringly supervised.
- If they understand what the stimuli will look like, how to respond, and how long the test will take.
- If they understand that the instrument will adjust its timing to their individual reaction time and pace, and that there is no need to rush.
- If they know that they can pause the test if they need to, by holding the response button down.

Patients and staff affect each other. Positive staff behavior creates positive patient attitudes, and vice versa. Failure to provide patients with important information and reassurance can exacerbate their fears about disease and blindness, and cause frustration with the process in general. Patient frustration also can lead to staff frustration—because staff tire of hearing patient complaints, and because frustrated patients tend to produce less useful visual field test results. In the end, positive staff and patient attitudes and behavior start with the doctor, as we now will discuss.

The attitude of the doctor is most important here. She or he can help ensure effective perimetry by explaining to the patients why perimetry is important in treatment decisions, and by supporting and instructing the perimetric staff.

Processes That Can Promote Success

THE DOCTOR'S ROLE

The doctor must explain and demonstrate to the patient why visual field testing is helpful (Fig 2-1). The doctor should explain to glaucoma patients that tonometry alone is not enough, and that what really counts is how well they see now and how well they will see in the future. Tell them that perimetry provides important indications of whether their current therapy is sufficient. You may show patients illustrative parts of their visual field test results, explaining again why this is useful information. In our experience patients who understand the value of perimetry and who have been properly coached during their initial tests will be quite willing and able to do visual field testing, and will require less staff and doctor attention in future perimetry tests.

We now know that technician training and motivation strongly affect visual field outcomes and that, with proper training, the frequency of testing artifacts can be reduced to low levels.[2] This is why we believe that doctors must periodically discuss with staff members how and why visual field testing should be performed, why it is important to carefully coach new patients, and that careful patient management can improve test result quality, patient compliance, and patient satisfaction. In

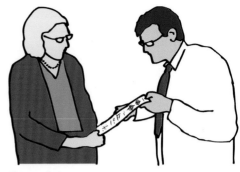

Figure 2-1

The doctor should explain the importance of visual field testing at least once to each patient undergoing routine perimetric testing.

some situations, it may be appropriate to delegate the training of new staff to experienced employees, but there can be no substitute for clear communication of positive attitudes and positive expectations by the doctors leading a practice.

THE ROLE OF THE PERIMETRIST

Entering patient identification data

It is crucial that some pieces of patient data be entered correctly. Most important is that the patient's name, date of birth, and identification number are always entered in the same way. This is a prerequisite for the perimeter to be able to automatically identify and analyze all of the patient baseline and follow-up tests. Date of birth is important, because it is used in age adjustment of the STATPAC normative data and also to optimize testing conditions.

An easy way to ensure that identification data are accurate and consistent is to recall the patient's name from previous tests using the perimeter's "Recall Patient Data" function. If you are using ZEISS FORUM software to connect your Humphrey perimeter to your office computer network, you can download patient data from the FORUM database, or in some cases from your electronic health record system (Fig 2-2).

Refractive correction

Refractive blur reduces visual sensitivity to perimetric stimuli, and it is standard practice to provide refractive correction using trial lenses when testing the central visual field. One diopter of refractive blur in an undilated patient will produce a little more than one decibel of depression of the hill of vision when testing with a Goldmann Size III stimulus.[3] Fully presbyopic patients are therefore provided with +3.25

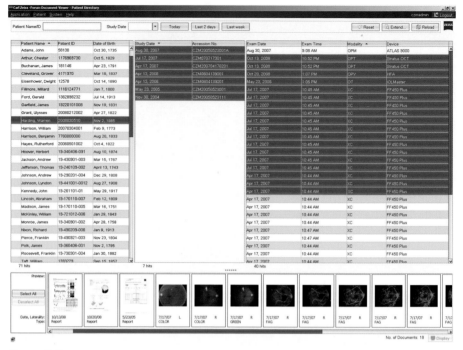

Figure 2-2

Downloading patient identification data from a FORUM database saves time and helps ensure correct and consistent entry of such information. This procedure helps ensure that all patient tests are available for progression analysis, etc. In this example identification data are being chosen for fictional patient Warren Harding.

diopter near additions relative to their distance refraction. Patients who are less than fully presbyopic are given lesser additions, either according to standard age-based correction tables programmed into the perimeter or based upon clinical judgment. Trial lens correction is only used when necessary for clear vision in central field testing, and is never used for testing outside of 30°.

In most testing situations, we prefer to leave cylindrical errors of less than 2 diopters uncorrected and instead to add the spherical equivalent to the spherical correction. The reason is that small astigmatic errors have little effect upon results, and the likelihood of trial lens artifacts increases considerably when a second lens is added.

The patient should be carefully aligned to the correction lenses. The pupil should be at the center of the lens, and the lens should be placed as close to the eye as possible without having the lashes touch it when blinking.

Instructing the patient

There is value in standardizing the instructions that patients receive. Much may be lost when the elements of what patients need to know are passed down from one perimetrist to the next. We prefer to maintain a standardized instruction message for perimetrists to refer to, even if they are not expected to always follow it verbatim (see chart).

The following instructions may be read to new patients, or may serve as a guide in defining your own standard instructions. Experienced patients will seldom need such detailed instruction, but new patients will produce more reliable tests and will be more relaxed if they hear and understand each of the points below.

PATIENT INSTRUCTIONS	PERIMETRIST
1. This test will measure the central and side vision of each eye individually. During the test, always look straight ahead at the steady yellow light.	Point to yellow fixation light.
2. Other lights will flash one at a time off to the side. Press the button whenever you see one of these lights.	Give patient the response button.
3. The test is designed so that it will dim the light flashes until you no longer can see them. Thus, you are not expected to see all the lights, and in fact you probably will see fewer than half of them. This also means that many of the lights you do see will be barely visible.	Explain procedure to patient.
4. If you want to pause the test, hold down on the button. The test will resume when you release the button.	Demonstrate to patient.
5. Testing time varies, but typically takes 5 minutes or more. You can blink normally. When your test is over, you will hear two beeps. You may then sit back and rest.	Explain procedure to patient.

Foremost in each new patient's mind will be two basic questions: What will the test be like and how long will it last? The perimetrist must explain and demonstrate to new patients what the stimulus will look like, where it might appear, that the test will take several minutes per eye, that blinks are allowed, how to sit, how to pause the test, and so on (Fig 2-3). For instance, patients should be told that they can blink as usual, and that they may temporarily pause the test by holding the response button down. Patients also should be reassured that there is plenty of time to respond—that the instrument will adapt to each patient's individual speed. Perimetrists should undergo threshold visual field testing in order to be better prepared to communicate this information.

New patients must clearly understand that when they see a light and press the button, that response is just a signal for the computer to later present a dimmer light at the same location. The aim of the test is to measure the limit of vision at many test point locations. Thus, in every threshold test more than half of the stimuli presented will be too dim to be seen, even for a person with perfect vision, and most of the stimuli that are seen are likely to be barely visible.

Patients may want to know how bright the light must be for them to press the button. We have found that the best answer to this question is that they should press the button if they believe that they have seen a stimulus.

Which eye to test first

Conventionally, the right eye usually is tested first. Recently, at least one study has found no testing order effect, suggesting that on the average it probably does not matter which eye is tested first.[4] Still, knowing that some patients may fatigue more than others, we continue to start with the right eye unless there is a reason to do otherwise, so that any fatigue effects will be as constant as possible from visit to visit.

Positioning the patient

Chair height and instrument height must be adjusted for patient comfort. Proper comfort is much more important in perimetry than, for instance, in slit lamp biomicroscopy, simply because perimetric examination takes longer and also because any discomfort is likely to distract the patient from the task at hand.

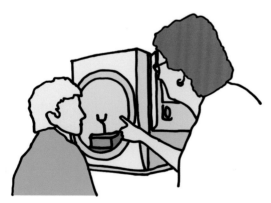

Figure 2-3
The perimetrist plays a central role in the success of visual field testing. Patients who are inexperienced in visual field testing will perform better and feel more comfortable if properly instructed and supported by the perimetrist. Experienced patients will need much less instruction and supervision, especially if they have received careful care on their first test.

Generally, we have found that patients are most comfortable if sitting more or less erect, preferably in an office chair that supports their arms. Having to lean forward into the instrument can cause the patient to place too much weight on the chin rest, which often becomes uncomfortable after just a few minutes. Leaning forward also requires an uncomfortable backward flexure of the neck in order to fit into the chinrest and headrest. We find it best to encourage an upright natural posture and to help the patient slide the chair up to the instrument so that upright posture is maintained. It may be helpful to note that in such an upright position, the patient's legs are under the perimeter, not out in front of the instrument (Fig 2-4).

Running the test

The perimeter has a demonstration mode that should be used before starting the "real" part of test in patients who are not yet experienced test takers. The demo test runs for 1 minute unless the perimetrist presses the Start Test button. It is not necessary to run the demo test for very long; often just a few seconds is enough. The perimetrist can simply press the Start Test button once it is clear that the patient has understood how to respond.

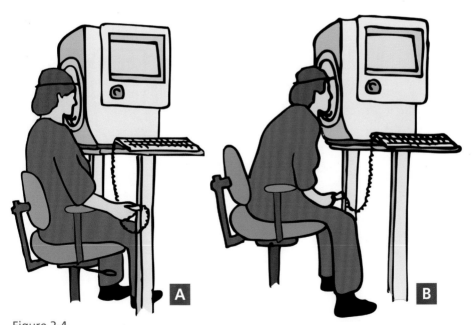

Figure 2-4
Patients usually are most comfortable if sitting more or less erect, with their legs well under the instrument (A). Leaning forward into the chin rest (B) tends to be uncomfortable and to cause neck and back strain.

In new patients, the perimetrist should be attentive and available during the test to answer questions and to reassure the patient. The perimetrist also must periodically check that the patient is still in proper position and aligned with the correction lens. Experienced patients will require considerably less supervision when they return for follow-up testing, as long as they have been carefully instructed and supervised during their first few tests.

Things to watch for during the test include:

- Does the patient seem reasonably comfortable, alert, and calm?
- Is the eye still centered behind the trial lens?
- Is the lens still close to the eye, or has the patient backed away from the headrest?
- Is the patient blinking from time to time?
- Is the patient looking straight ahead at the fixation light?
- Is the upper eyelid high enough so that the pupil is not blocked?
- Is the patient's head reasonably straight, or has it become tilted to the right or left?
- Is the chair still in the right position, or has it slid back from the perimeter?

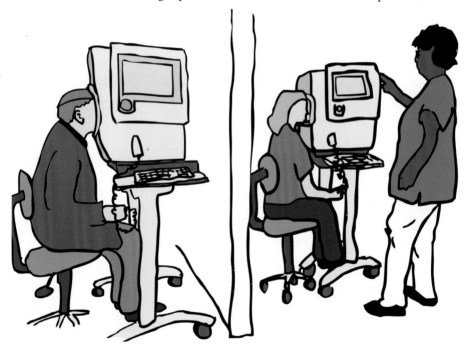

Figure 2-5
In clinics having several perimeters, it often makes sense to place all instruments in the same room, sometimes separated by partitions, or at least curtains. One perimetrist can then supervise more than one patient at the same time.

Experienced patients generally need much less supervision and it is quite possible for one technician to manage several experienced patients and perimeters at the same time if the testing environment has been suitably organized[5, 6] (Fig 2-5). The HFA has a video output port that allows installation of a duplicate screen in another room. The remote screen will show the same information that is being presented on the perimeter's video screen.

An optional feature on some HFA models automatically senses the position of the patient's pupil and adjusts the chin rest and forehead rest in tiny (0.3 mm) steps—right-left, and up-down—with the goal of keeping the eye centered relative to the trial lens. An optional automatic vertex distance monitor also sounds an audible alarm if the patient backs away from the lens holder. These features are intended as adjuncts to proper patient instruction and supervision and not as replacements.

3

Basic Principles of Perimetry

COMPUTERIZED PERIMETRY IS most effective when the user is familiar with the basic principles underlying its operation and use.

Normal and Abnormal Visual Fields

The normal field of vision extends more than 90° temporally, 60° nasally and superiorly, and about 70° inferiorly, but most diagnostic visual field testing concentrates on the area within 30° of fixation, where most retinal ganglion cells are located. Visual sensitivity is greatest at the very center of the field and decreases toward the periphery. The visual field is commonly represented as a hill, or island of vision (Fig 3-1). The height or sensitivity of the normal hill of vision is affected by age, the general level of ambient light, stimulus size, and stimulus duration.

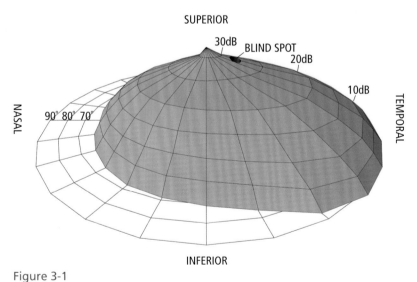

Figure 3-1

Hill of vision for the right eye of a normal 51-year-old person tested with a Size III stimulus. Vision normally extends more than 90° temporally and less in other directions. The height of the hill represents sensitivity, which is highest at the point of fixation and gradually decreases towards the periphery. Most clinical testing is done in the central visual field, within 30° of fixation.

The types of visual field defects most commonly seen in different diseases will be discussed later. For the moment it should simply be said that a field defect is any statistically significant depression of sensitivity compared to the normal hill of vision. Alternatively, a visual field defect might be defined as any decrease in peripheral vision that is unusual among normal subjects. Estimates of statistical significance of threshold sensitivity findings are provided by the STATPAC analysis program of the Humphrey perimeter (Chapter 5). Field defects may be localized or general, and localized defects may also be combined with general depression of the whole field. Localized field defects can be described in terms of both size and depth, and quantification of such defects is diagnostically helpful. An area of the visual field where the patient still has some remaining vision but where sensitivity is less than normal is called a relative defect, while an area where the maximum available stimulus is not seen is termed an absolute defect.

A generally depressed field without localized loss is a nonspecific finding and is usually caused by cataract, miosis, or lack of proper refractive correction during the test. Field defects that are quite evident on perimetric test results usually are not perceived by the patient. This is due to the so-called "filling-in" effect[7-10] (Fig 3-2). This is why patients seldom tell us about symptomatic visual field loss and why we must rely upon visual field testing to detect such damage.

Applications of Perimetric Findings

This book primarily addresses the application of perimetry to diagnosis and therapeutic decision-making. The goal of perimetry in such cases is to obtain information important to diagnosis and to the therapeutic decision at hand, and perimetric testing is directed toward those portions of the visual field that are most likely to be informative about the presence or stability of a particular disease. Such examinations generally involve careful measurement of light sensitivity at various locations in the field. Because light sensitivity is commonly defined as the minimum perceivable brightness, the term "threshold sensitivity" usually is used.

Perimetry may also be used to determine the extent of remaining visual function for insurance purposes or in order for the patient to qualify for a driver's license. In such instances, subtle defects often are ignored. Most commonly, these examinations are performed by presenting bright stimuli at various locations throughout the tested area—a brightness that would not be missed unless there were rather profound losses of vision.

Computerized Static Perimetry

Computerized static perimetry has been the clinical standard of care since the mid-1980s. Over the years a number of researchers have reported computerized static perimetry to be superior to various methods of carefully performed manual perimetry.[11-16]

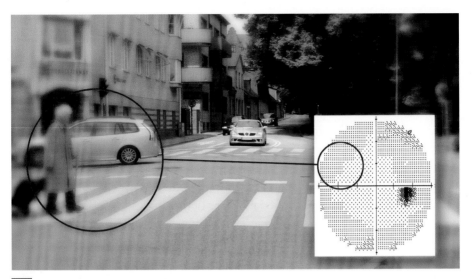

A

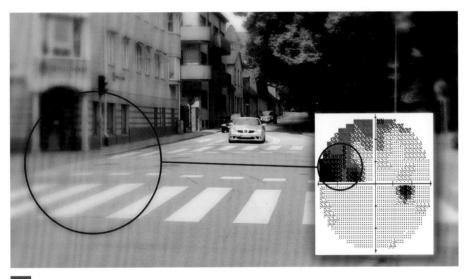

B

Figure 3-2

Most field defects are negative scotomas, which means that they will not be perceived, for instance as darker or blurred areas. Instead the brain will cause so-called "filling-in" creating an inaccurate but "believable" image in the part of the patient's visual field that is defective. A patient with a nasal field defect may therefore fail to see the pedestrian and the car shown in (A) (seen by a normal eye) but instead perceive a "believable" image of the intersection such as that shown in (B). Note that both the normal and the damaged visual field simulations illustrate the lower resolution that is typical of peripheral vision compared to central vision.

Computerized threshold static perimetry involves measuring the differential light sensitivity at a number of predetermined test point locations. Static perimetry was performed manually long before computers were widely available,[17] but because of the complexity of the technique and the difficulty of keeping track of multiple patient responses, the method was used only in a few research settings. Computerization made it possible to automate thresholding algorithms and to keep track of patient responses at all of the points under examination. Improvements in computer processor speed later facilitated the development of increasingly complex, and increasingly efficient, methods of data acquisition, as well as data analysis methods that previously had been impractical in clinical care.

Another important benefit of computerization is that it enabled standardized testing, which has greatly improved test comparability between clinics and around the world. Indeed, standardization in perimetry now is so highly valued that most clinics and hospitals have standardized on Humphrey perimetry and a narrow range of testing procedures—most commonly a 24-2 SITA threshold test.

Issues in Instrument Design

A basic perimeter might be characterized as an instrument that can project a stimulus of known size and intensity onto a screen or background having a known brightness for a known amount of time at a known location in the visual field. Effective visual field testing can be achieved only if each of these factors is carefully controlled.

STIMULUS SIZE AND INTENSITY

The Humphrey perimeter presents white light stimuli that can be varied in brightness over a range of 5.1 log units (51 decibels [dB]) between 0.08 and 10,000 apostilbs (asb). The decibel (dB) value refers to stimulus intensity, with 0 dB corresponding to the maximum brightness that the perimeter can produce (10,000 asb) and 51 dB corresponding to 0.08 asb (Fig 3-3). In standardized testing with a Size III white stimulus, the dimmest stimulus that can be seen by a young, well-trained observer is a little less than 40 dB. Thus, the upper (and dimmest) 10 dB of the stimulus range— from 41 to 51 dB—really fall outside the range of human vision under standard testing conditions.

Threshold sensitivity is determined in Standardized Automated Perimetry (SAP) by varying only the stimulus brightness, not stimulus size. The Humphrey perimeter is capable of testing with the five standard Goldmann stimulus Sizes (Fig 3-4), but the 0.43 degree Goldmann Size III stimulus is used almost exclusively. Size V is sometimes employed in advanced field loss, while the Sizes I, II, and IV are almost never used in static visual field testing.

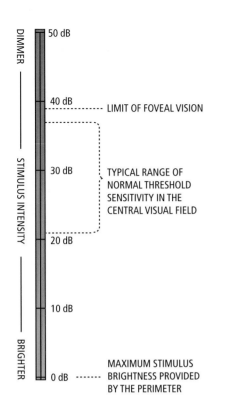

DIMMER — STIMULUS INTENSITY — BRIGHTER

50 dB

40 dB ----------- LIMIT OF FOVEAL VISION

30 dB ⁞ TYPICAL RANGE OF
NORMAL THRESHOLD
SENSITIVITY IN THE
CENTRAL VISUAL FIELD

20 dB

10 dB

0 dB ------ MAXIMUM STIMULUS
BRIGHTNESS PROVIDED
BY THE PERIMETER

Figure 3-3
Visual field sensitivity is measured and expressed in decibels (dB), which is a logarithmic unit. Under standard testing conditions the maximum sensitivity found in healthy, young, normal subjects is a little under 40 dB. The maximum stimulus brightness of the perimeter (10,000 apostilbs) corresponds to 0 dB.

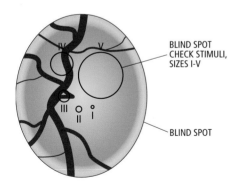

BLIND SPOT
CHECK STIMULI,
SIZES I-V

BLIND SPOT

Figure 3-4
Goldmann test spot sizes I through V are available in the Humphrey Field Analyzer (HFA). All test targets are much smaller than the physiological blind spot, which normally measures approximately 5° horizontally by 7° vertically. Spot sizes differ in angular subtense by factors of two, with Sizes I through V subtending 0.1°, 0.21°, 0.43°, 0.86°, and 1.72°, respectively.

BACKGROUND ILLUMINATION

In standard Humphrey perimetry, stimuli are projected onto a surface that itself is uniformly illuminated at a brightness of 10 Cd/m^2 (31.5 apostilbs). This background illumination brightness was originally used by the Goldmann perimeter and is an internationally recognized standard.[18] This adaptation level was chosen because it approximates the minimum brightness for photopic, or daylight, vision—vision that depends upon retinal cone function rather than on rods. The advantage of testing the photopic visual system is that visibility depends more on object contrast and less on absolute brightness. Under photopic testing conditions, changes in pupil size or crystalline lens color and transparency have less effect on test results. At dimmer, scotopic levels of retinal adaptation, absolute object brightness becomes more important than contrast, and pupil size and media effects become more difficult to control.

STIMULUS DURATION

The Humphrey perimeter uses a standard stimulus duration of 200 milliseconds (ms), which is long enough for visibility to be little affected by small variations in duration, but still shorter than the latency for voluntary eye movements, so the patient does not have time to see the stimulus in the peripheral visual field and then look toward it.

STIMULUS LOCATION AND FIXATION MONITORING

Accurately mapping visual field sensitivity requires knowledge of where on the retina each stimulus is presented. While it is not difficult to calibrate where the instrument itself shows the stimulus, knowledge of where the patient is looking at the moment of stimulus presentation is less precise. Fortunately, most patients fixate adequately, and the problem of proper stimulus location has primarily become one of identifying those few patients whose gaze is so unsteady that they should be reinstructed on proper fixation technique.

The gaze tracker on the Humphrey perimeter measures gaze direction with a precision of about 1° and automatically records gaze direction each time a stimulus is presented. Gaze tracking results are shown on the video screen during testing and are presented at the bottom of the test printout.[19]

The original Humphrey perimeter relied upon the Heijl-Krakau blind spot monitoring technique[20] rather than a gaze tracker. This method provided an index of the quality of patient fixation during an examination by periodically presenting stimuli in the blind spot. Positive responses were presumed to indicate poor fixation. See Chapter 5 for further discussion on fixation monitoring.

Threshold Testing

The objective of static threshold perimetry is to measure the differential light sensitivity at each tested location. Such findings always are subject to some variability because of variabilities in the visual system itself, as well as occasional patient mistakes. Successful testing strategies balance time efficiency with provisions to account for such uncertainties.

Humphrey threshold strategies start testing at a single location in each quadrant of the visual field (Fig 12-4). If a stimulus is seen, subsequent stimuli at that location are dimmed one step at a time until no longer seen. Conversely, if the initial stimulus is not seen, then subsequent presentations are made brighter in steps until the patient presses the response button. Some strategies repeat this process for confirmation of the finding, either using the same brightness step size, or perhaps a smaller increment.

For efficiency, the threshold finding at each quadrant's first tested point is used to determine the initial brightness at adjacent points, and so on. Test pacing—the time interval between stimuli—is determined by measuring patient response time.

Suprathreshold Testing

Suprathreshold testing and threshold testing have different goals. Suprathreshold testing is intended to establish whether or not sensitivity is abnormally low at any location in the visual field. Because a suprathreshold test presents the patient with fairly bright stimuli that should be seen if vision is reasonably normal, it is easy to use with patients who have never been tested before.

Historically, suprathreshold tests were much shorter than the early threshold tests, but this speed advantage was considerably reduced with the availability of SITA Fast 24-2 testing. Suprathreshold tests also do not provide quantitative data, and are not as sensitive to early field loss as threshold tests.[21] As a result, suprathreshold testing is used much less often now than in the early days of automated perimetry. Nevertheless, one should remember that suprathreshold tests are easier for inexperienced patients and therefore may still have a role in patients in whom the suspicion of field loss is small, for example in patients having a positive family history of glaucoma but no other suspicious findings.

Kinetic Perimetry

Kinetic perimetry was the standard method of clinical visual field testing until the mid-1980s. A stimulus of known size and brightness was slowly moved from the periphery toward the center of the field, until the patient reported seeing it. The point where the stimulus was detected was noted and the same stimulus was brought in from different angles around the hill of vision. Connecting all the points where the stimulus first was detected produced an isopter. The test was continued using other stimulus brightness and/or sizes until enough isopters had been produced to characterize the shape of the hill of vision. Analysis of test results was done in a qualitative manner, as normative data and statistical analysis packages were not available.

Today, kinetic perimetry has largely been replaced by automated static perimetry. However, kinetic testing still may be required in some institutions or in some countries for disability certification, and in some specialized diagnostic situations. The Humphrey perimeter is capable of performing kinetic testing, and instructions may be found in the most current User Manual.

4

Choosing a Test

W HEN A PERIMETRIC TEST is needed, a 24-2 Size III white SITA Standard threshold test usually is the best choice. This chapter explains why this is so, and then discusses the exceptions to this rule.

Choosing a Test Pattern

The Humphrey Field Analyzer (HFA) 30-2 test pattern measures visual sensitivity at 76 locations within 30° of fixation—the area commonly referred to as the central visual field. The 24-2 test pattern consists of the 54 most central test locations of the 30-2 pattern (Fig 4-1). Over the years, the 24-2 test pattern has become more generally used than the 30-2, because little diagnostic information is lost,[22, 23] and considerable testing time is saved compared to the 30-2. Fewer trial lens and lid artifacts also are seen with the 24-2 test pattern. One argument in favor of the 30-2 test pattern is that progression can sometimes be found earlier, simply because more locations are tested.[24]

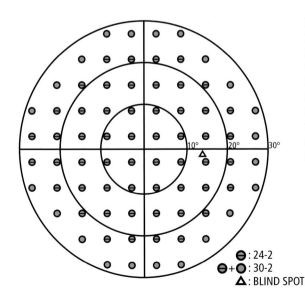

Figure 4-1
Point locations making up the 24-2 test pattern are a subset of those in the 30-2 test pattern. Essentially, a 24-2 test is just a 30-2 with all of the outer ring of test points removed, except for the nasal-most two. Test points are spaced 6° apart. These are the patterns for a right eye.

⊖: 24-2
⊖+●: 30-2
▲: BLIND SPOT

Central versus Peripheral Testing

Most visual field tests are ordered in connection with the diagnosis or management of glaucoma, and the standard of care in glaucoma management concentrates on testing the central field. A few early glaucoma patients will first present with field loss outside the central 30° only,[25, 26] but since this occurs infrequently and since the range of normal peripheral sensitivity is quite large, peripheral field testing is rarely done in glaucoma management.

Even in neurological disease, most of the diagnostic information is in the central field.[27, 28] Thus, the 30-2 and 24-2 test point patterns are the preferred standards also for neurological visual field testing. There are a few exceptions. One such exception could be when a small central scotoma is suspected in a patient having normal or near-normal visual acuity but a history suggesting acute optic neuritis. Then a 10-2 test with foveal threshold will provide a denser 2-degree grid spacing with a higher number of test points in the very central visual field (Fig 4-3). The 10-2 test also is valuable when evaluating visual field loss in macular disease.

Occasionally, peripheral testing is done to rule out retinal detachments, or to differentiate between detachment and retinoschisis in eyes that cannot be well visualized ophthalmoscopically, but this is the exception rather than the rule (see Chapter 11).

Choosing Stimulus Size

Computerized static perimetry has established the Goldmann white, Size III stimulus as standard. Therefore, normative data and statistical analysis packages for standard perimetry using white stimuli are based upon the Size III stimulus. See the Exceptions section of this chapter for a discussion of when a nonstandard stimulus size might be advantageous.

Choosing a Test Strategy

The patented SITA thresholding strategies[29-31] available on Humphrey perimeters are about twice as fast as the older strategies they replaced.[32-42] SITA Fast takes about two-thirds the time of SITA Standard, and a few healthy and highly experienced subjects have been able to complete SITA Fast 24-2 testing in less than 2 minutes. While we prefer SITA Standard for most testing situations, we believe that SITA Fast offers similar performance to SITA Standard, but with somewhat larger test-retest variability.[40]

Early strategies stopped testing at each test point based on firmly fixed criteria, either the crossing of threshold a single time, a second time, or even a third and fourth time. SITA strategies gain efficiency by ceasing testing when predetermined statistical levels of testing certainty are reached, rather than when specific numbers of stimuli or threshold crossings have occurred. This method allows test time to be shortened when reliably consistent responses are given, and extended when there still is uncertainty;[29] the primary difference between the SITA Standard and SITA Fast strategies is the amount of certainty that is required before testing can be stopped. The overall effect usually is reduced testing time without loss of diagnostic information.

Thus, the SITA strategies have clear advantages over conventional methods and should be used whenever available. We recommend use of SITA Standard because it is more precise even though not as quick as SITA Fast (Fig 4-2). SITA Fast is less tolerant of patient mistakes and may best be used in experienced or younger patients. SITA Fast presents stimuli that more often are just barely visible, and may be a more difficult test than SITA Standard. Therefore, SITA Fast is not the preferred choice in patients expected to have difficulty with perimetric testing.

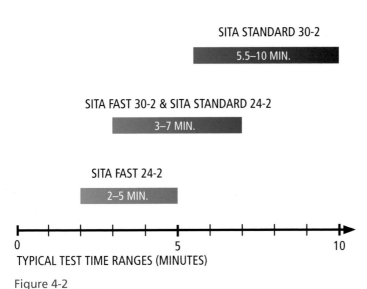

Figure 4-2
Typical ranges of test times for the most commonly used HFA tests. Test times are shorter in normal fields and longer in abnormal fields.

Exceptions

While most Humphrey perimetric examinations are performed using a SITA 24-2 or 30-2 threshold testing, a number of less common clinical presentations can occur that call for alternative approaches.

LATE STAGE GLAUCOMA

In the very late stages of glaucoma when mainly central islands of vision remain, one can switch to a SITA Standard or SITA Fast 10-2 test, which covers only the area within 10° of fixation using a grid of test points spaced every 2° (Figs 4-3 and 4-4A–B). Another possibility is to use the larger Size V stimulus, with a 30-2, 24-2, or 10-2 pattern (Fig 4-4C–D). Using a Size V stimulus will extend the available sensitivity range, often making it possible to continue following patients with very advanced field loss. However, nonstandard stimulus sizes cannot be used with the SITA testing strategies and you will no longer have access to normative data or the Humphrey Guided Progression Analysis.

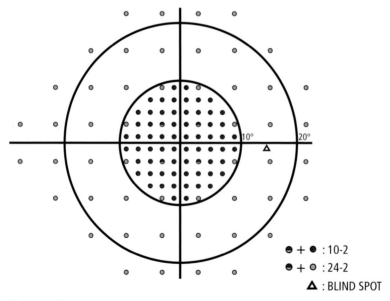

Figure 4-3
The 10-2 test point pattern shown in red provides a detailed image of the most central field, i.e., the visual field within 10° of fixation. Here, the 10-2 pattern is compared with the more generally used 24-2 test pattern shown in blue. The 10-2 test may be useful, e.g. in advanced glaucoma, or when mapping the visual field in patients with age-related macular degeneration. The spacing between test points is 2°. This is the pattern for a right eye.

TESTING FOR DRUG-INDUCED MACULOPATHIES

Patients undergoing long-term treatment with hydroxychloroquine or similar medications are frequently sent for ophthalmic consultation in order to monitor for drug-associated maculopathy. New guidelines now emphasize the importance of automated imaging, electroretinogram, and fundus autofluorescence in monitoring for toxicity. Nevertheless, 10-2 white automated perimetric examination remains part of the recommended regimen.[43] At the time of publication of this edition, the American Academy of Ophthalmology recommendations emphasized the importance of investigating even slight losses in the central 10-2 visual field. Use of red stimuli has been advocated by some, but no clear advantages have been documented compared to standard white stimulus testing, and normative limits for red testing are not available.

DISABILITY TESTING

Perimetric testing to determine visual disability may be performed for a number of reasons, for instance to determine eligibility for insurance compensation, to facilitate rehabilitation in patients with visual impairment, to establish fitness to drive, and sometimes to document the need for blepharoplasty. Regardless of the purpose, disability testing requires a different approach from that used in standard diagnostic perimetry. The goal in diagnostic perimetry is to detect changes that indicate early disease or to document measured progression, or sometimes improvement. In disability testing, the goal is to identify profound visual dysfunction; thus tests for disability usually are performed using strong stimuli that will be missed only if there is clear, well-defined damage. The stimulus most commonly used for such tests is the Goldmann III 4e stimulus, which in Humphrey terms is Size III, 10 dB white. Such a stimulus often is used in a single-level, suprathreshold testing mode, since threshold testing takes longer and adds no important information in these applications.

Insurance Eligibility

Standards for perimetric assessment of disability insurance eligibility vary from country to country, and, in some countries, from one government agency to the next. The US Social Security Administration (SSA) recently endorsed use of a new criterion for disability determinations, stating that an MD of −22 dB on a 30-2 Humphrey threshold visual field corresponds approximately to a constriction of the visual field to less than 20° from fixation, and recommending an MD of worse than 22 dB as a visual field criterion to define disability.[44]

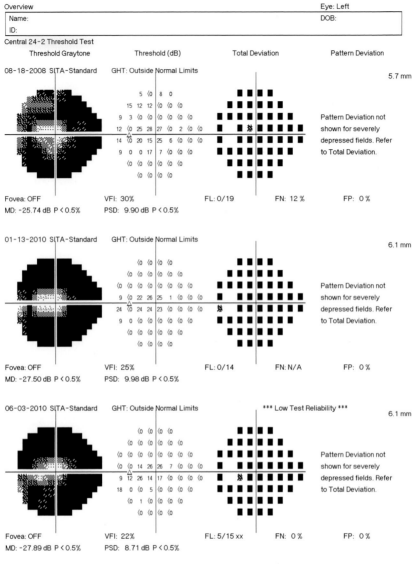

Figure 4-4

In very late stages of glaucoma where only a few points in the 24-2 or 30-2 patterns have remaining vision (A and C), one might switch to a Swedish Interactive Thresholding Algorithm (SITA) 10-2 test (B). In some cases it might be more useful to switch to a Size V stimulus but continue using the 24-2 or 30-2 pattern (D).

Overview   Eye: Left

Name:	DOB:
ID:	

Central 10-2 Threshold Test

Threshold Graytone	Threshold (dB)	Total Deviation	Pattern Deviation

09-27-2011 SITA-Standard   6.3 mm

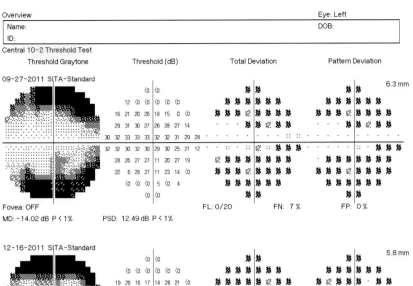

Fovea: OFF   FL: 0/20   FN: 7 %   FP: 0 %

MD: -14.02 dB P < 1%   PSD: 12.49 dB P < 1%

12-16-2011 SITA-Standard   5.8 mm

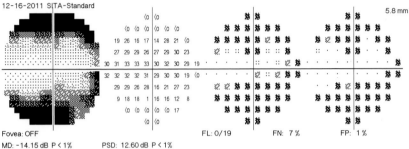

Fovea: OFF   FL: 0/19   FN: 7 %   FP: 1 %

MD: -14.15 dB P < 1%   PSD: 12.60 dB P < 1%

02-24-2012 SITA-Standard   5.7 mm

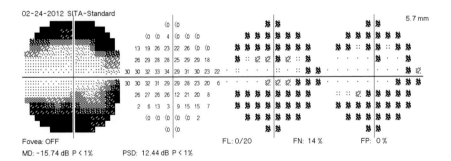

Fovea: OFF   FL: 0/20   FN: 14 %   FP: 0 %

MD: -15.74 dB P < 1%   PSD: 12.44 dB P < 1%

:: < 5%
✾ < 2%
✾ < 1%
■ < 0.5%

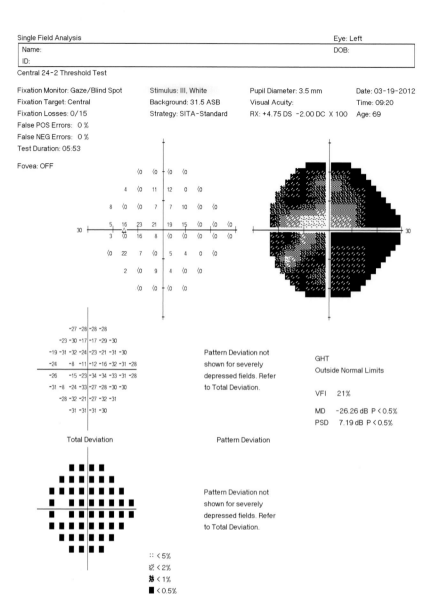

Single Field Analysis | Eye: Left
Name: | DOB:
ID:

Central 24-2 Threshold Test

Fixation Monitor: Gaze/Blind Spot
Fixation Target: Central
Fixation Losses: 0/15
False POS Errors: 0 %
False NEG Errors: 0 %
Test Duration: 05:53

Fovea: OFF

Stimulus: III, White
Background: 31.5 ASB
Strategy: SITA-Standard

Pupil Diameter: 3.5 mm
Visual Acuity:
RX: +4.75 DS −2.00 DC X 100

Date: 03-19-2012
Time: 09:20
Age: 69

Total Deviation

Pattern Deviation not
shown for severely
depressed fields. Refer
to Total Deviation.

Pattern Deviation

GHT
Outside Normal Limits

VFI   21%

MD   −26.26 dB P < 0.5%
PSD   7.19 dB P < 0.5%

Pattern Deviation not
shown for severely
depressed fields. Refer
to Total Deviation.

:: < 5%
※ < 2%
※ < 1%
■ < 0.5%

Figure 4-4
continued

Name:	DOB:
ID:	

Central 24-2 Threshold Test

Fixation Monitor: Gaze/Blind Spot	Stimulus: V, White	Pupil Diameter: 3.5 mm	Date: 03-19-2012
Fixation Target: Central	Background: 31.5 ASB	Visual Acuity:	Time: 09:30
Fixation Losses: 0/21	Strategy: FASTPAC	RX: +4.75 DS -2.00 DC X 100	Age: 69
False POS Errors: 0/13			
False NEG Errors: 1/13			
Test Duration: 11:56			

Fovea: OFF

Threshold Graytone

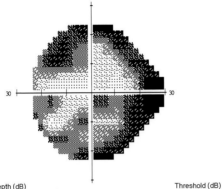

30   30

Defect Depth (dB)

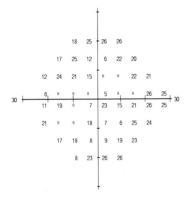

```
                18   25  | 26  26
            17  25   12  |  6  22  20
        12  24  21   15  |  0   0  22  21
     6   0   0   0  |  5   0   0  26  25
30 ─┼──────────────┼──────────────┼─ 30
    11  19   0   7 | 23  15  21  26  25
        21   0   0  18  |  7   6  25  24
            17  18   8  |  9  19  23
                 8  23  | 26  26
```

Threshold (dB)

    176   165

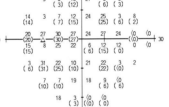
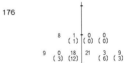

```
                    8     1  | 0    0
                       ( 1) |( 0) ( 0)
                  9     0   18 | 21    3    9
                     ( 3) (12) |    ( 6) ( 3)
            14     3    7   12 | 24   25    3    8
          (14)  ( 7) (15) |   (25) ( 6) ( 2)
            20    27   30  27 | 24   27   24   <0  <0
          (20)─△─(30)─(27)┤                 (<0
30 ─┼──────────────┼──────────────┼─ 30
            15     8   25  22 |  6   12   12   <0  <0
          (15)              |  ( 6) (15) ( 0)    (<0
             3    31   22   10 | 21   22    3    2
          ( 6) (31) (25) (10) |    ( 6) (22) (<0)
             7     7   19 | 18    9   <0
          (10) (10) |        ( 6) ( 6)
                   18    3  | <0   <0
                       ( 3) |(<0) ( 0)
```

    196   100

0 = Within 4 dB of Expected

Central Reference: 30 dB xx

The Esterman test is one of the methods commonly used in disability testing, and binocular and monocular versions of this test are offered as standard testing options on current Humphrey perimeters (Fig 4-5). The Esterman test is performed using the patient's customary distance spectacles, without making any near refractive addition; the goal being to take into account whatever visual field limitations might be imposed by the spectacles, and the assumption being that the stimuli used are so strong as to not be much affected by any refractive blur associated with the near testing distance.

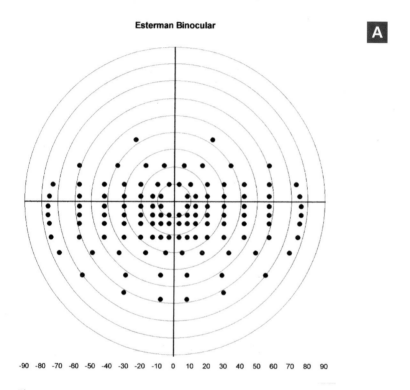

Figure 4-5

The Esterman Binocular test (A) is commonly used for disability testing, or as in this case (B–D) driver's license qualification. The field defects of the two glaucomatous fields (C–D) do not overlap much, and therefore few stimuli have been missed on the Esterman Binocular test (B).

| Name: | DOB: |
| ID: | |

Esterman Binocular

Fixation Monitor: OFF   Stimulus: III, White   Pupil Diameter: Date: 01-26-2009
Fixation Target: Central   Background: 31.5 ASB   Visual Acuity: Time: 16:14
Fixation Losses: 0/0   Strategy: Two Zone   RX: DS   DC X   Age: 60
False POS Errors: 5/10 xx   Test Mode: Single Intensity
False NEG Errors: 0/10
Test Duration: 04:23

Stimulus Intensity: 10 dB

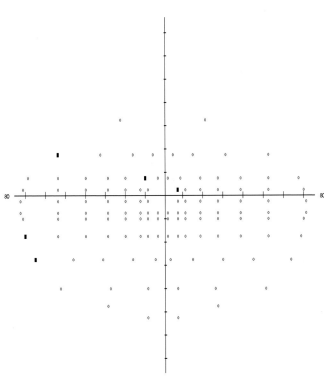

∘ Seen 115/120
▪ Not Seen 5/120
△ Blind Spot
Esterman Efficiency Score: 95

Name:
ID:

Eye: Right
DOB:

C

Central 30-2 Threshold Test

Fixation Monitor: Gaze/Blind Spot
Fixation Target: Central
Fixation Losses: 2/21
False POS Errors: 8 %
False NEG Errors: 0 %
Test Duration: 09:11

Fovea: OFF

Stimulus: III, White
Background: 31.5 ASB
Strategy: SITA-Standard

Pupil Diameter: 5.1 mm
Visual Acuity:
RX: +0.50 DS   DC X

Date: 09-22-2008
Time: 10:47
Age: 60

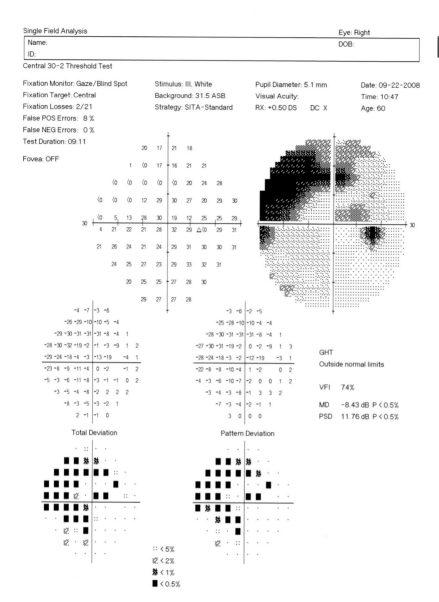

GHT
Outside normal limits

VFI   74%

MD   -8.43 dB P < 0.5%
PSD   11.76 dB P < 0.5%

Total Deviation

Pattern Deviation

:: < 5%
▨ < 2%
▩ < 1%
■ < 0.5%

Figure 4-5
continued

Single Field Analysis

Eye: Left

Name:	DOB:
ID:	

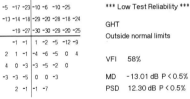

D

Central 30-2 Threshold Test

Fixation Monitor: Gaze/Blind Spot

Fixation Target: Central

Fixation Losses: 8/21 xx

False POS Errors: 13 %

False NEG Errors: 6 %

Test Duration: 10:42

Fovea: OFF

Stimulus: III, White

Background: 31.5 ASB

Strategy: SITA-Standard

Pupil Diameter: 4.6 mm

Visual Acuity:

RX: +0.00 DS   DC X

Date: 09-22-2008

Time: 10:57

Age: 60

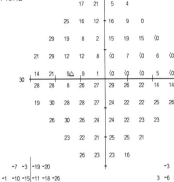

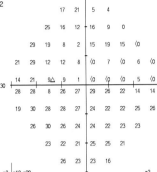

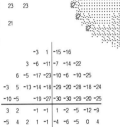

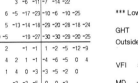

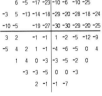

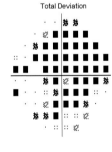

Total Deviation

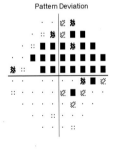

Pattern Deviation

*** Low Test Reliability ***

GHT

Outside normal limits

VFI   58%

MD   -13.01 dB P < 0.5%

PSD   12.30 dB P < 0.5%

:: < 5%

▨ < 2%

⚹ < 1%

■ < 0.5%

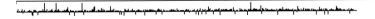

Driving

Automobile drivers' licensing is sometimes based partially upon visual field assessment. In many jurisdictions such assessment is the exception rather than the rule, and no internationally accepted standards now exist. The overall binocular visual field is most important in driving, and losses in one eye may be well compensated for by the other eye.[45] Eye movement can also compensate somewhat for binocular field loss, but the patterns of eye movements seem to be different in patients with bilateral visual field defects as compared to healthy individuals when viewing a traffic scene.[46]

Anderson et al. have suggested that, in the absence of more conservative guidelines from local authorities, drivers should have binocular visual fields extending at least 50° both to the right and to the left of fixation.[47] The authors do not provide any suggestions regarding the superior and inferior fields except to note that overhead objects such as traffic signals usually do not require an extensive superior visual field, at least when viewed from a distance.

Blepharoptosis

Perimetry is frequently used to document visual impairment secondary to blepharoptosis, although nonperimetric methods also may be used.[48–50] Such testing is best done using single-level suprathreshold testing and a bright stimulus. It may be helpful to recall that it is quite common, especially in elderly patients, to find asymptomatic and apparently nondisabling field restrictions affecting the upper row of test points of the central 30° visual field caused by the eyelid. Thus, it may not be necessary to test outside the central visual field when investigating the effects of blepharoptosis.

SWAP

Short wavelength automated perimetry (SWAP), also known as blue-yellow perimetry, is a specialized technique in which blue Goldmann Size V stimuli are presented on a bright (100 Cd/m²) yellow background. The yellow background serves to reduce the responsiveness of the red and green cone systems so that the blue stimuli are seen primarily by the blue cone system.

For many years SWAP was believed to allow earlier detection of glaucomatous visual field loss than conventional white-on-white perimetry.[51, 52] However, more recent research has not been able to confirm these findings, and, on the contrary, it now appears that SITA testing with standard white stimuli may detect just as much field loss in glaucoma as SWAP, [53] and also at least as early.[54]

Because of SWAP's higher test-retest variability and larger sensitivity to cataract, we no longer recommend SWAP for glaucoma management. In the future SWAP may instead find a place in managing patients with diabetic retinopathy.[55-57]

OTHER COLORED STIMULI

We are frequently asked whether colored stimuli should be used in automated static perimetry. We are aware of no evidence showing that colored stimuli on a white background offer any advantages over standard white stimuli, and since no normative data exist for such stimuli, they are almost never used. See the section on drug-induced maculopathies earlier in this chapter.

5

STATPAC Analysis of
Single Fields

S TATPAC IS A GROUP of computerized analysis packages included in the operating system of the Humphrey perimeter, consisting primarily of the STATPAC Single Field Analysis (SFA) and the Guided Progression Analysis (GPA2).[58-60] STATPAC simplifies and standardizes the analysis and presentation of visual field test results, in order to help practitioners at all levels of perimetric experience come to more consistent and, we believe, more useful assessments of test results.[61]

The STATPAC SFA compares results of a single threshold test with age-corrected normative data, and highlights findings that deviate significantly from normal (Fig 5-1). The SFA also presents indices of test reliability, and raw test results. This chapter will focus on assessment of the results from a single field test. See Chapter 6 for a discussion of how to detect and quantify change over time.

Newer and older Humphrey threshold testing strategies (SITA Standard, SITA Fast, SITA SWAP, Full Threshold, and Fastpac) all give slightly different threshold test results. STATPAC uses different normal limits for the different strategies, and probability printouts and analyses like the Glaucoma Hemifield Test and Glaucoma Change Probability Maps all present results that are applicable to the specific test used, and are based on large and separate collections of normative data for each strategy. The two most frequently used test patterns, 30-2 and 24-2, are based upon the same normative limits, except that the limits for MD and PSD (which are discussed later in this chapter) in the 24-2 test pattern are calculated just from the 24-2 test points. The SITA 10-2 normative data were collected separately and are not based upon the 24-2/30-2 normals data.

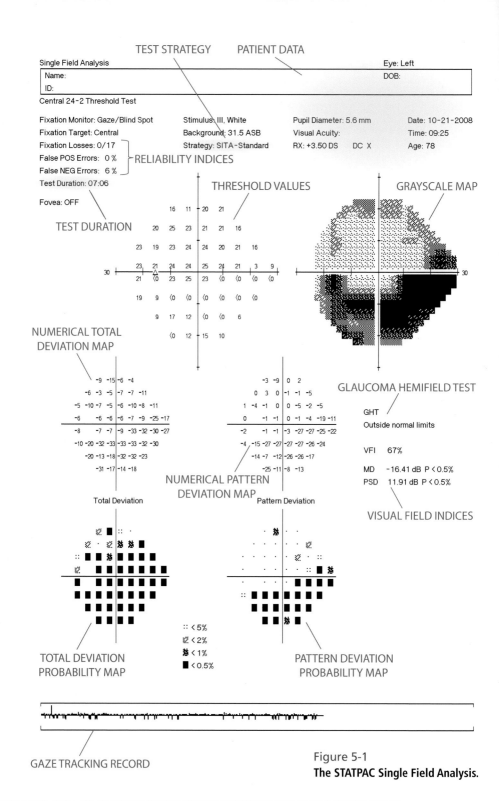

Figure 5-1
The STATPAC Single Field Analysis.

Information Presented on the
Single Field Analysis (SFA) Report

DEMOGRAPHICS AND TESTING CONDITIONS

Patient name, identification number, date of birth, age, the date and time of testing, visual acuity, pupil size, and eye tested all are presented at the top of the SFA printout.

TOTAL DEVIATION

Total Deviation probability plots identify test locations that are outside normal limits. Threshold sensitivity is compared with the age-corrected normal values at each test point to produce the Total Deviation (TD) numerical map. The statistical significances of these deviations from normal depend upon test point location and the test strategy used, and are indicated in the associated Total Deviation probability plot, in which deviations are highlighted when they are worse than those found in the bottom 5%, 2%, 1%, and 0.5% of sensitivities in normal subjects of the same age as the patient. A key showing the meaning of the symbols is given near the bottom of the printout. A 2% symbol, for instance, indicates that 98% of normal subjects of the same age would be expected to have a sensitivity that is higher than the recorded value.

The range of sensitivity found among healthy subjects is larger in the periphery than in the center of the field. Thus, a deviation of 5 dB from age-normal sensitivity is quite unusual—and therefore statistically significant—at the center of the field, but is totally within the normal range of sensitivity in the periphery of the test area.

PATTERN DEVIATION

The single most useful analysis on an SFA printout is the Pattern Deviation (PD) probability plot. The Pattern Deviation analysis shows sensitivity losses after an adjustment has been made to remove any generalized depression or elevation of the overall hill of vision. The PD plot uses the same symbols as the Total Deviation plots to identify points deviating by statistically significant amounts from the range of values typically found in healthy subjects.

Cataract causes generalized depression, which can complicate detection of localized early glaucomatous defects. By removing the generalized component of field change, the Pattern Deviation analysis can highlight subtle localized loss while largely ignoring cataract effects.

The strength of the probability maps is that they ignore results that are within normal variability and highlight subtle, but statistically significant, variations that might otherwise escape notice (Fig 5-2). Probability maps also help deemphasize

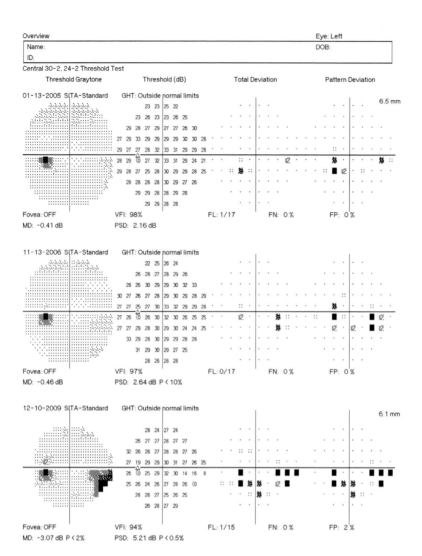

Name: DOB:
ID:

Central 30-2, 24-2 Threshold Test

| Threshold Graytone | Threshold (dB) | Total Deviation | Pattern Deviation |

01-13-2005 SITA-Standard   GHT: Outside normal limits   6.5 mm

Fovea: OFF   VFI: 98%   FL: 1/17   FN: 0%   FP: 0%
MD: -0.41 dB   PSD: 2.16 dB

11-13-2006 SITA-Standard   GHT: Outside normal limits

Fovea: OFF   VFI: 97%   FL: 0/17   FN: 0%   FP: 0%
MD: -0.46 dB   PSD: 2.64 dB P < 10%

12-10-2009 SITA-Standard   GHT: Outside normal limits   6.1 mm

Fovea: OFF   VFI: 94%   FL: 1/15   FN: 0%   FP: 2%
MD: -3.07 dB P < 2%   PSD: 5.21 dB P < 0.5%

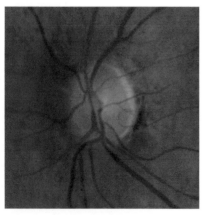

Figure 5-2

Subtle abnormalities often are considerably more distinct in probability maps than on grayscale maps. Thus, it is common to see developing field loss appear earlier in probability maps than in grayscale maps (A), in this case in an eye with rather subtle disc abnormalities (B).

common artifactual patterns, such as eyelid-induced depressions of sensitivity in the superior part of the field, that often appear on the grayscale (Fig 12-2). Artifactual field loss is discussed in Chapter 12.

COMPARING TOTAL DEVIATION AND PATTERN DEVIATION

It is useful to compare the Total Deviation and Pattern Deviation maps when evaluating clinical cases. If the two maps look more or less the same, then there is little or no generalized depression. On the other hand, a uniformly depressed Total Deviation map combined with a normal-looking Pattern Deviation map probably indicates a cataract (Fig 5-3). The opposite pattern—a Pattern Deviation map that looks more disturbed than its corresponding Total Deviation map—often is associated with a trigger-happy patient who has repeatedly pressed the response button when no stimulus was seen (Figs 5-4 and 12-5).

GLAUCOMA HEMIFIELD TEST

The Glaucoma Hemifield Test (GHT) provides a plain language classification of 30-2 and 24-2 test results based upon patterns of loss commonly seen in glaucoma.[62, 63] Pattern Deviation scores in each of five zones in the upper hemifield are compared to findings in mirror-image zones in the inferior visual field. Scoring differences between mirror image zones are compared to normative significance limits specific to each zone pair (Fig 5-5).

GHT findings are divided into the following categories:

- "Outside Normal Limits" is displayed whenever at least one zone pair differs by an amount found in fewer than 1% of normal subjects.

- Fields not classified as Outside Normal Limits are labeled as "Borderline" whenever at least one zone pair differs by an amount found in fewer than 3% but more than 1% of normal subjects.

- "General Depression" or "Abnormally High Sensitivity" messages are presented whenever even the best test point locations are either so low or so high as to be at levels seen in fewer than half a percent of normal subjects.

- The "Within Normal Limits" message is presented whenever none of the above conditions are met.

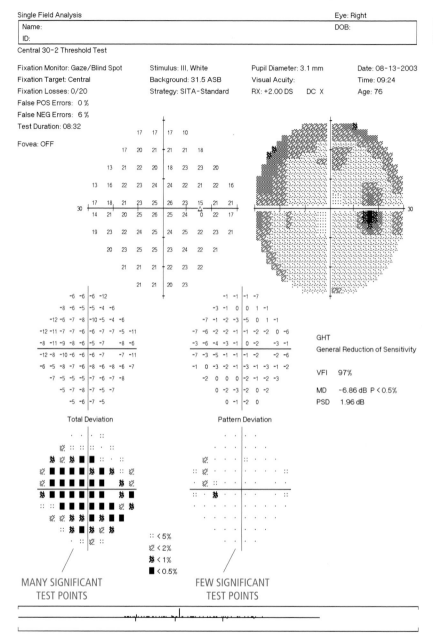

Figure 5-3

A typical cataract pattern with a considerably greater number of significantly depressed test point locations in the Total Deviation probability map than in the Pattern Deviation probability map (A). After surgery (B) the two probability maps are much more similar.

Single Field Analysis   Eye: Right

Name:	DOB:
ID:	

Central 30-2 Threshold Test

Fixation Monitor: Gaze/Blind Spot	Stimulus: III, White	Pupil Diameter: 3.0 mm	Date: 03-01-2005
Fixation Target: Central	Background: 31.5 ASB	Visual Acuity:	Time: 09:26
Fixation Losses: 0/17	Strategy: SITA-Standard	RX: +2.25 DS DC X	Age: 77

False POS Errors: 0 %

False NEG Errors: 3 %

Test Duration: 07:07

Fovea: OFF

```
                20  21  20  18
            21  24  25   24  24  23
        17  24  25  26   26  26  27  24
    14  24  24  27  28   28  27  27  27  20
    18  23  25  28  29   29  28  21  26  24
30  19  24  26  29  31   30  30  10  26  26   30
    19  23  25  28  29   29  29  30  27  24
        18  23  26  27   28  28  27  25
            22  27  24   26  27  27
                22  22   24  24
```

Total Deviation

```
          -2  -1 | -2  -4
      -4  -1  -1 | -1  -1  -1
   -9  -3  -3  -3 | -2  -2   1  -2
 -10 -3  -5  -3  -3 | -2  -2  -2   0  -6
  -8  -5  -5  -3  -2 | -2  -2      -2  -3
  -6  -5  -5  -2  -1 | -2  -1      -2  -1
  -6  -5  -4  -3  -2 | -2  -2   0  -1  -4
   -8  -5  -4  -4 | -2  -2  -2  -4
      -5  -1  -5 | -3  -2  -1
          -4  -5 | -3  -3
```

Pattern Deviation

```
          -1   0 | -1  -3
      -3   0   0 |  0   0   0
   -7  -2  -2  -1 | -1  -1   2  -1
  -9  -2  -4  -2  -1 | -1  -1  -1   1  -5
  -6  -4  -4  -2  -1 | -1  -1      -1  -2
  -5  -4  -4  -1   0 | -1   0      -1   0
  -5  -4  -3  -2  -1 | -1  -1   1   0  -3
   -7  -4  -3  -2 | -1   0  -1  -3
      -4   0  -4 | -2  -1   0
          -3  -4 | -2  -2
```

GHT
Within normal limits

VFI   99%

MD   -2.87 dB P < 2%

PSD   1.98 dB

Total Deviation

Pattern Deviation

:: < 5%

▨ < 2%

▩ < 1%

■ < 0.5%

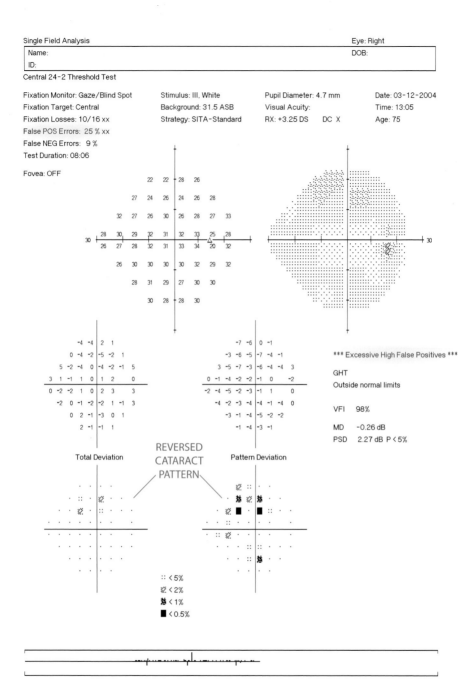

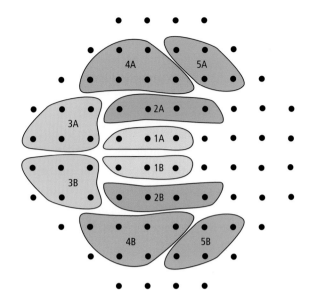

Figure 5-5
The Glaucoma Hemifield Test (GHT) compares Pattern Deviation probability scores in five zones in the upper field with corresponding mirror image zones in the lower hemifield. Statistically significant findings produce plain language messages on test reports. All points used are common to both the 24-2 and 30-2 test point patterns.

The GHT has been reported to have high sensitivity and specificity,[64] and the user who is still getting used to visual field interpretation may find identifying glaucomatous visual field loss on the basis of GHT findings to be the best choice. The method was designed to have an overall target specificity of approximately 94% when Borderline findings are treated as being within normal limits, and about 84% when Borderline findings are considered outside normal limits. Actual specificity will depend upon the clinical population being examined. Highly experienced users should expect to find that they sometimes prefer their own interpretations to those offered by this analysis. Note that the GHT's zone pattern is designed to be sensitive to glaucomatous visual field damage. It was not designed to be sensitive to field loss caused by diseases other than glaucoma, such as neurological field loss.

GLOBAL INDICES

Three summary indices of visual field status—VFI, MD, and PSD—appear on the SFA printout.

VFI (Visual Field Index) is a recently developed staging index, designed to be less affected by cataract and also to provide improved correspondence to ganglion cell loss compared to MD.[60] VFI is approximately 100% in normal fields and approaches 0% in perimetrically blind fields.

MD (Mean Deviation) shows how much on average the whole field departs from age-normal, and is a center-weighted average of the decibel deviations shown in the Total Deviation plot. MD is primarily used to stage visual field loss and as a metric for rate of change over time. MD is approximately 0 dB in normal fields and –30 dB to –35 dB in extreme visual field loss, depending upon patient age and test program.

PSD (Pattern Standard Deviation) reflects irregularities in the field, such as those caused by localized field defects. PSD is small, close to zero, both in normality and in blindness, and peaks at moderate levels of localized field loss; because of this nonlinear behavior, PSD should not be used as a staging or progression index.

RAW TEST RESULTS: GRAYSCALES AND NUMERIC PRINTOUTS

Simple threshold sensitivities measured at each test point are presented both in numerical and grayscale form. Sensitivities are indicated in decibels (dB), which are tenths of a log unit; 0 dB indicates a test point location where only the maximum available stimulus brightness (10,000 asb) was seen; 10 dB indicates a stimulus one-tenth as bright (1,000 asb); 20 dB one hundredth of maximum brightness (100 asb), and so on. A 40 dB (1 asb) stimulus is slightly fainter than the foveal threshold sensitivity of most young perimetrically experienced subjects.

RELIABILITY INDICES

Three indices are presented to assist in the evaluation of test reliability. They estimate the rates of false positive response errors, false negative response errors, and fixation loss errors.

False Positive Response Errors

The false positive (FP) response error score measures the tendency of patients to press the response button even when no stimulus has actually been seen— in order to identify so-called trigger-happy patients. With the SITA strategies, patient responses that are made at impossible or unlikely times are used to estimate FP response rates. These include responses made before or during stimulus presentation, or too soon after stimulus presentation, considering patient reaction times measured during the same test. Because FP rates depend strongly upon assessment of patient reaction time over the whole course of the test, the FP rate is not calculated until after testing has been completed.

The FP index is the most important and useful of the three available reliability indices. We find FP rates exceeding 15% to be strongly associated with compromised test results, and usually it is best to repeat such tests. See Chapter 12 for examples of test results having excessive FP rates. Tests having FP rates exceeding 15% are automatically removed from GPA analyses (Chapter 6).

False Negative Errors

The false negative (FN) error score was originally meant to assess patient inattention—and to help identify patients who have failed to respond to stimuli that probably should have been seen. FN rates are measured by occasionally presenting very bright stimuli at test point locations where threshold sensitivity already has been found to be reasonably normal. A problem is that FN rate estimates are elevated in glaucomatous visual field tests, even in highly attentive patients (Fig 5-6). Thus, the FN index is of limited utility in glaucoma management and high FN rates in glaucomatous fields should not be blamed on the patient, but are a characteristic of the glaucomatous eye.[65-69]

Fixation Loss Rate

The fixation loss (FL) rate measures patient gaze stability—whether the patient is gazing straight ahead or looking from side to side during the test. FL rates are estimated by periodically presenting stimuli at the presumed location of the patient's blind spot—the so-called Heijl-Krakau method.[20] Positive patient responses to such stimuli suggest that the patient may not be looking straight ahead. Because the normal blind spot is approximately 5° or 6° in diameter, fixation shifts of approximately half of that amount—about 3°—can be detected.

FL rates exceeding 20% may suggest compromised test results. However, high FL levels frequently are seen artifactually, such as when the blind spot has not been properly located, in trigger-happy patients, or because patients have been allowed to tilt their heads enough that the blind spot check stimulus falls on normal retina instead of on the blind spot.

Another disadvantage of this method is that fixation checks add to the test time and therefore can be made only occasionally during the test. Because of this low data density and the frequent artifactual findings mentioned above, we prefer to turn off FL catch trials and to rely upon the HFA's full-time gaze tracker (see below).

GAZE TRACKING

In most Humphrey perimeters, an automatic dual-variable gaze tracker measures gaze direction every time a stimulus is presented. A record of gaze stability is presented at the bottom of the SFA printout. In most patients, measurements are precise to approximately ± 1°.

Single Field Analysis   Eye: Right

Name:	DOB:
ID:	

Central 30-2 Threshold Test

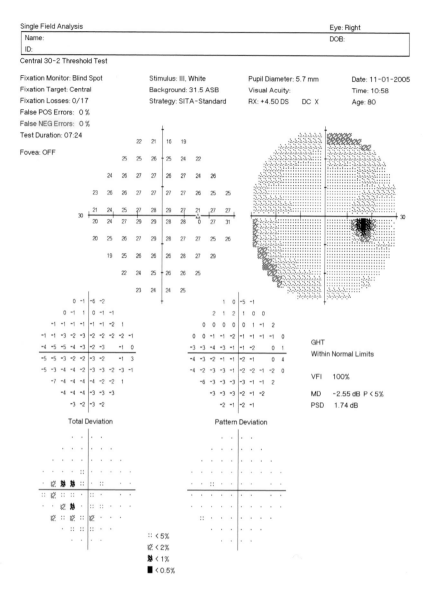

Fixation Monitor: Blind Spot   Stimulus: III, White   Pupil Diameter: 5.7 mm   Date: 11-01-2005
Fixation Target: Central   Background: 31.5 ASB   Visual Acuity: Time: 10:58
Fixation Losses: 0/17   Strategy: SITA-Standard   RX: +4.50 DS   DC X   Age: 80
False POS Errors: 0 %
False NEG Errors: 0 %
Test Duration: 07:24
Fovea: OFF

GHT
Within Normal Limits

VFI   100%

MD   -2.55 dB P < 5%
PSD   1.74 dB

Total Deviation

Pattern Deviation

:: < 5%
▨ < 2%
▩ < 1%
■ < 0.5%

Figure 5-6

The percentage of false negative answers tends to be higher in abnormal glaucomatous fields than in normal fields. This often is obvious in patients with unilateral glaucoma. In this patient there were 0% FN answers in the normal right eye (A), but 13% false negative errors in the glaucomatous left eye (B). In general, a field test showing considerable glaucomatous field loss should not be discarded simply because it has a high percentage of FN, nor should the patient be reinstructed or retested.

Name:	DOB:
ID:	

Central 30-2 Threshold Test

Fixation Monitor: Blind Spot
Fixation Target: Central
Fixation Losses: 1/23
False POS Errors: 1 %
False NEG Errors: 13 %
Test Duration: 10:41

Fovea: OFF

Stimulus: III, White
Background: 31.5 ASB
Strategy: SITA-Standard

Pupil Diameter: 4.7 mm
Visual Acuity:
RX: +3.75 DS -2.25 DC X 28

Date: 11-01-2005
Time: 11:07
Age: 80

```
                ⟨0   5    4   12
           6   11   ⟨0   18  16  19
      ⟨0  ⟨0   ⟨0   21   19  20   6  17
  11  ⟨0  ⟨0   ⟨0    2   19  21  22  19  17
    9   6   0   17   21  26  22  23  20   8
30                                          30
   20  21  ⟨0   23   21  12  ⟨0  18   3   2
   22  13  24   20   ⟨0  ⟨0  ⟨0   7  ⟨0   5
      14  15   14    8  ⟨0   9  15   6
          ⟨0   11    9   20   3   0
                7   19   19   5
```

```
      -23 -17 -18 -10                        -15 -9 -10 -2
    -18 -14 -27 -8  -9  -6                  -10 -6 -19  0  -1   2
  -27 -28 -29 -6  -9  -8 -21 -8           -19 -20 -21  2  -1   0 -13  0
-15 -29 -30 -31 -28 -11 -8  -7  -8  -7    -7 -21 -22 -23 -20 -3  0   1  0   1
-18 -22     -13 -10 -5  -8  -7  -8 -17    -10 -14    -5 -2  3  -1   1  -1  -9
 -8  -8      -8 -10 -19 -33 -13 -25 -23    0   0      0 -2 -12 -25 -5 -18 -15
 -5 -15 -5 -10 -33 -33 -33 -23 -30 -20    3  -7   3  -2 -25 -25 -25 -15 -22 -12
  -14 -14 -16 -22 -32 -21 -13 -21          -6  -6  -8 -14 -24 -13 -5 -13
    -30 -18 -19 -8 -24 -26                  -22 -10 -12 -1 -17 -18
      -20 -8  -7 -21                         -12  0   1  -13
```

GHT
Outside Normal Limits

VFI   58%

MD   -17.48 dB P < 0.5%
PSD   10.92 dB P < 0.5%

Total Deviation

Pattern Deviation

:: < 5%
▨ < 2%
▩ < 1%
■ < 0.5%

On the gaze tracking record, lines extending upward indicate the amount of gaze error during each stimulus presentation, with full scale indicating gaze errors of 10° or more. Lines extending downward indicate that the instrument was unsuccessful in measuring gaze direction during that particular stimulus presentation, for instance, because of a blink. Guidelines for interpretation of gaze tracker results are shown in Fig 5-7.

The HFA's gaze tracker uses image analysis to separately locate the center of the pupil and the reflection of a light emitting diode from the corneal surface. The spacing between these two features strongly depends upon gaze direction while being largely independent of changes in patient head position. Separate calculations provide head position information that is used in one model of the HFA to automatically keep the eye aligned at the center of the trial lens. At the time of this writing, the HFA was the only commercially available perimeter having such a dual variable gaze tracking system.

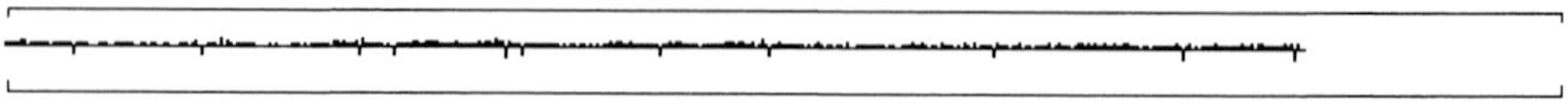

Figure 5-7: Gaze Tracker A
Exemplary fixation stability, with no gaze errors of any significant magnitude

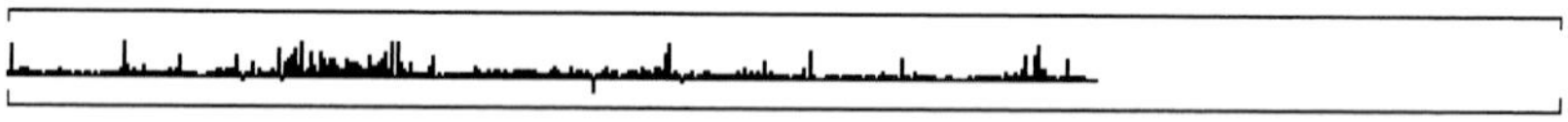

Figure 5-7: Gaze Tracker B
Mostly consistent fixation, except for a period of instability about a quarter of the way into the test. Field showed a well-defined area of abnormality that was consistent with follow-up tests and the result was considered to be of good reliability.

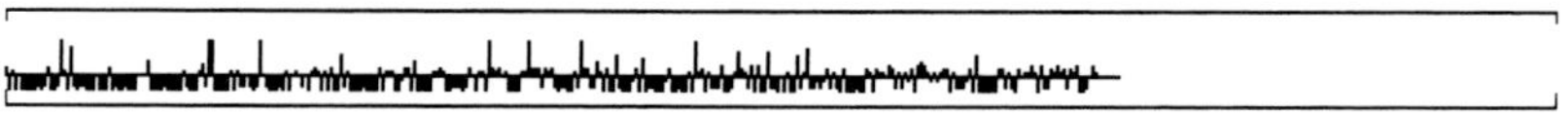

Figure 5-7: Gaze Tracker C
Frequent loss of tracking signal caused by blinks or other interference by the lids or lashes is indicated by the many downward deflections in the trace, and may have been caused by ptosis. Sometimes it is helpful to use surgical tape to hold the eyelid up and out of the way.

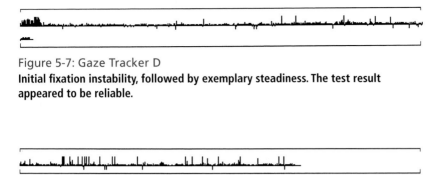

Figure 5-7: Gaze Tracker D
Initial fixation instability, followed by exemplary steadiness. The test result appeared to be reliable.

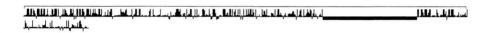

Figure 5-7: Gaze Tracker E
Occasional gaze track errors. This represents good fixation stability.

Figure 5-7: Gaze Tracker F
Unreliable fixation. Numerous maximal gaze errors are combined with loss of tracking signal late in the test.

6

Assessing Perimetric Change

OPHTHALMIC AND NEUROLOGICAL DISEASE can cause significant visual field changes, and assessment of those changes over time can help practitioners decide whether or not a patient is recovering, stable, or getting worse. Visual field changes that are both statistically and clinically significant may provide a basis for adjustments in prognosis or therapy. However, because increasingly aggressive therapies often have increased side effects and risks, therapeutic escalation decisions may also depend upon whether or not the observed rate of change poses a threat to the patient's quality of life.[70, 71]

Measurement of Visual Field Progression in Glaucoma

Standard Automated Perimetry (SAP) plays a central role in glaucoma management, simply because the primary effect of glaucomatous progression is continued loss of visual function. Standardized progression analysis increases the level of agreement between practitioners[72] and can help quantify the amount of progression found.

The most widely available analysis aid for quantifying visual field progression is the Humphrey perimeter's Guided Progression Analysis, or GPA. GPA helps doctors identify and quantify visual field progression in glaucoma patients, using both event and trend analysis. Event and trend analyses have different but complementary goals. The goal of event analysis is to assess whether there has been any statistically significant worsening in the visual field. The goal of trend analysis is to quantify any observed rate of change, and to help the practitioner assess the risk of future visual disability associated with that rate. Our preferred report for use in glaucoma management is the GPA Summary Report (Fig 6-1), which shows two baseline fields an event analysis of the most recent test, and a trend analysis of all available tests. However, if you wish to see event analyses of all available follow-up tests you may refer to the Full GPA report (Fig 6-2).

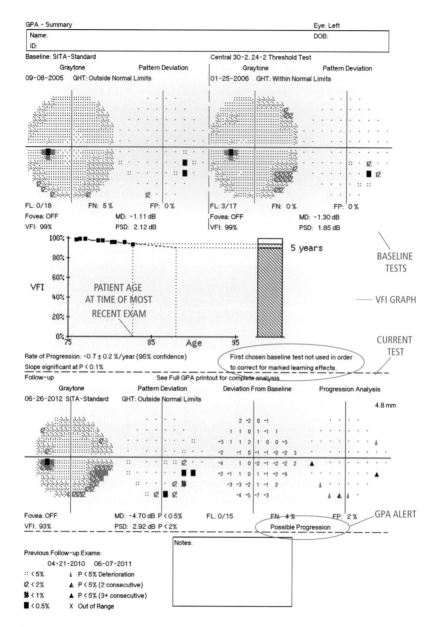

Figure 6-1

The Summary Report of the Guided Progression Analysis (GPA) is our preferred report for glaucoma management. This Summary shows two baseline fields at the top and the current field at the bottom. Both the Glaucoma Change Probability Map (an event analysis—see GPA EVENT ANALYSIS on page 67) and the Visual Field Index (VFI) graph (a trend analysis—see GPA TREND ANALYSIS on page 70) also are displayed. Patient age is shown on the x-axis of the VFI graph. This eye shows slow progression over 7 years of follow-up. Note that there was sufficient improvement between the first and second visual fields so that the GPA analysis used the second and third fields as baseline.

GPA EVENT ANALYSIS

The GPA's Glaucoma Change Probability Maps (GCPMs) are used as an aid in determining whether or not statistically significant progression has occurred. GPA provides a plain language event analysis called GPA Alert, which applies the progression criteria used in the Early Manifest Glaucoma Trial (EMGT) to GPA's Glaucoma Change Probability Maps.[73]

GPA Alert will display the message "Possible Progression" when three or more test points show statistically significant deterioration on two consecutive follow-up examinations, compared to a baseline of two field tests. A "Likely Progression" message will appear when the same three or more significantly deteriorated test points appear in at least three consecutive follow-up tests (Fig 6-2).

Analyses using the EMGT criteria have been reported to be both sensitive and specific compared to expert analysis. EMGT criteria have been reported to have a sensitivity of 96% compared to expert consensus. Mean time to detect progression was 33 months for EMGT, compared to 55 months and 66 months for two other analysis methods that had been used in other large-scale clinical trials. EMGT specificity was reported to be 89% for complete series of fields consisting of more than 20 tests, suggesting that specificity for analysis of 3 follow-up tests must be considerably higher. Analysis of only the points contained in the 24-2 test pattern decreased sensitivity to 91% but increased specificity for the whole series of more than 20 examinations to 96%. Median time to detect progression increased marginally using 24-2 points, from 33 months to 37 months.[24]

In a separate study, in cases of disagreement with GPA, expert consensus classification usually was that progression had occurred,[74] further confirming the high specificity of this analysis and suggesting that progression identified using the EMGT criteria probably has high credibility. However, GPA analysis requires at least 2 baseline and 3 follow-up tests, and users typically ordering perimetry for patients, for instance, only once a year should realize that in that setting a positive GPA progression result has high validity, while true progression may occur before the GCPM analysis has a chance of detecting it, since examination frequency is low.

The GPA's Change Probability Maps are based upon significance limits for change in Pattern Deviation,[59] and thus were designed to minimize the effects of cataract. Given the high incidence of cataract in the age group most likely to have glaucoma, we believe that such a strategy provides the high levels of specificity that are needed

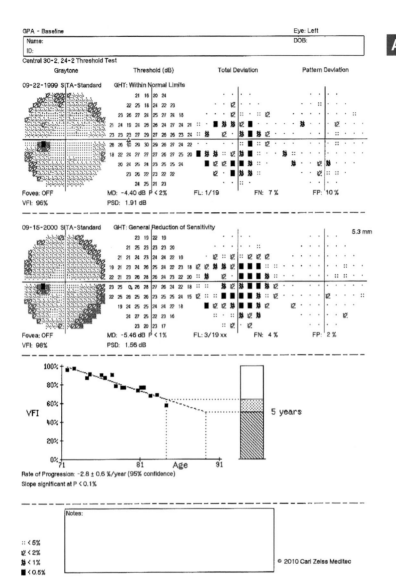

Figure 6-2

The Full GPA report displays the two baseline fields and the VFI analysis on page one (A). All eligible follow-up tests are shown in chronological order, plus a statement on each test stating whether statistically significant progression has been detected or not. The criteria for detecting progression are such that "Possible progression" is only displayed if the same three or more deteriorated test point locations have been identified on two consecutive follow-up tests (B). The "Likely progression" message is displayed only if statistically significant worsening as compared to baseline has been seen in the same three or more test point locations on three consecutive follow-up tests (C). Therefore, a finding of "Possible progression" requires that four tests are available (two baseline tests and two follow-up tests), and "Likely progression" requires a minimum of five tests.

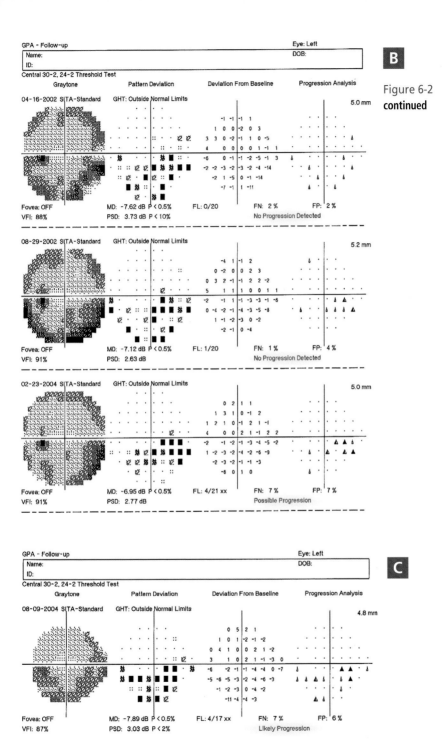

Figure 6-2
continued

in clinical glaucoma care and trials. However, this approach has been reported to be less sensitive than alternative methods in detecting conversion from ocular hypertension to very early glaucomatous field loss,[75] and analyses like the Glaucoma Hemifield Test continue to play a significant role in managing such patients.

GCPMs highlight test points deteriorating by more than the random variability typically found in perimetrically experienced glaucoma patients. GCPMs are based upon the variability observed in hundreds of glaucoma patients who were tested four times in the space of a month in an international multicenter clinical trial.[76] GCPMs also take advantage of detailed empirical knowledge developed over a 20-year period that quantifies how test-retest variability depends upon general field status, local defect depth, and test point eccentricity (Fig 6-3).[77] All these factors are included in the mathematical model that provides the basis for GCPMs.[59]

GCPMs use triangle symbols to highlight statistically significant deterioration from a baseline consisting of the average of two chosen tests. Each follow-up field is

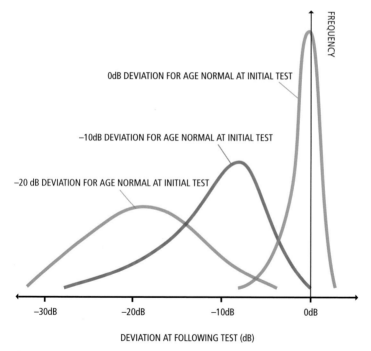

Figure 6-3
Random test-retest variability in glaucomatous fields is complex but has been characterized empirically in a multicenter clinical trial in order to produce the HFA's Guided Progression Analysis. Normal test points vary little, just a few decibels up or down (blue curve). Test point locations with damage and reduced sensitivity show larger variability (green and orange curves). Peripheral test points show higher variability than central test points.

compared to that baseline, and open triangles indicate test point locations with deterioration that is statistically significant at the 5% level. Half-black triangles indicate test point locations that have shown statistically significant deterioration in two consecutive follow-up examinations, and filled-in black triangles designate locations where such deterioration has been observed in three or more consecutive tests (Fig 6-4).

While GPA has been programmed to automatically choose two baseline tests after first looking for unreliable results and possible learning effects (Chapter 12), it still is good practice for the practitioner to confirm at least once that the automated choices are appropriate. The authors generally try to avoid choosing a baseline consisting of two quite different fields, or fields that have been taken several years apart. We recommend that the clinician review the instrument's choice of baseline tests when GPA analysis first is done. The user is free to manually select any two baseline fields, as long as the tests were done using the same testing strategy and as long as neither has a false positive response rate larger than 15%. It is probably not necessary to perform this review at every visit, as the GPA software has been programmed to remember and use the chosen baseline in subsequent follow-up tests. However, the practitioner should establish a new baseline after any major change in therapy, such as trabeculectomy, using two reliable and representative fields taken near the time when the change was made.

When evaluating Glaucoma Change Probability Maps the user should expect that each test point will have a 5% risk of being falsely flagged, simply from random test variability. The important lessons here are that 1) fields that truly are worsening will show reproducible change, and 2) credible change must be seen at multiple test point locations.[78] GCPMs are not calculated for fields having an MD value worse than −20 dB. This is because the mathematical model for calculating Pattern

   P < 5% Deterioration

   P < 5% (2 consecutive)

   P < 5% (3+ consecutive)

X   Out of Range

Figure 6-4
Symbols used in Glaucoma Change Probability Maps. The first time that a test point location shows statistically significant deterioration compared to baseline, it is marked with a narrow open triangle. At the next follow-up test, if the same point again shows significant worsening compared to baseline, the black and white triangle is displayed. If this result is confirmed at a third test, a filled black triangle is shown. Thus, the symbols become more visible as results become more significant. Some narrow open deterioration triangles are expected from chance alone.

Deviation, which forms the basis for the GCPMs, cannot be reliably applied when severe visual field damage is present.

GPA TREND ANALYSIS

The goal of trend analysis is to quantify how quickly each patient is changing and thereby to help doctors identify patients who are progressing at rates that threaten to cause considerable visual disability within the patient's expected lifetime (Chapter 8). Our preferred approach is to estimate rate of progression (ROP) using linear regression analysis of the Visual Field Index (VFI) over time.[60] This regression analysis is automatically displayed in the GPA Summary and the Full GPA reports whenever a sufficient number of visual field tests is available.

VFI is a single number that summarizes each patient's visual field status as a percentage of the normal age-corrected sensitivity. Thus, a completely normal visual field would have a VFI of 100%, and a perimetrically blind visual field—in which even the perimeter's brightest stimuli could not be seen—would have a VFI of 0%. VFI was designed to approximately reflect retinal ganglion cell loss. Thus, VFI gives central test points considerably more weight than peripheral ones, in order to better account for the much higher density of ganglion cells that is normally found in the central retina (Figs 6-5 and 6-6).

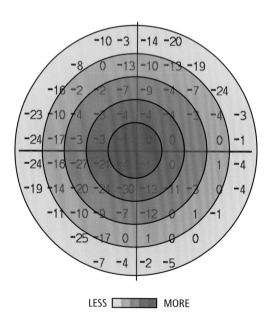

Figure 6-5
When calculating VFI, central test points are given much higher weight than peripheral ones, because of the much higher ganglion cell density closer to the center of the retina.

LESS ▭▬▬ MORE

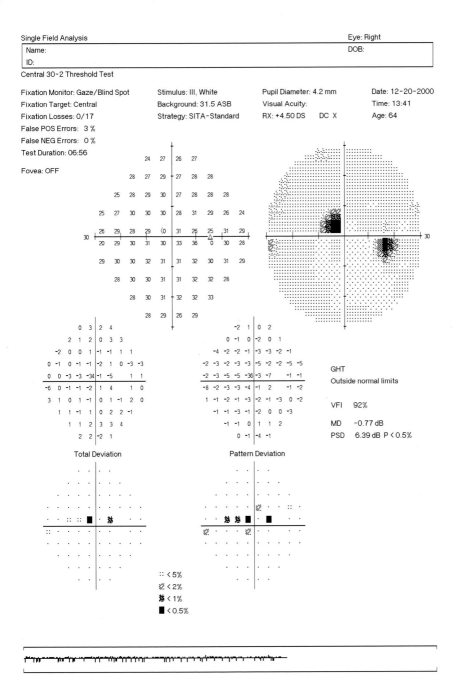

Figure 6-6

The high weight of central points in the VFI calculation is evident in this field with a single severely depressed test point location close to the point of fixation. The VFI value is reduced by 8% as compared to an age-corrected normal, while the Mean Deviation (MD) value is depressed by only 0.77 dB, or about 2.5%.

In the middle of each patient's GPA Summary Report is a graph displaying one VFI value for each reliable examination, plotted versus patient age (Fig 6-7). When at least five examinations are available, GPA performs a linear regression analysis on the plotted VFI values and calculates the patient's rate of progression in percent loss per year, along with the confidence limits for the slope estimate.

GPA provides a projection of the linear regression line into the future, if five or more exams covering at least 2 years are available, and if the width of the calculated 95% confidence interval for VFI slope is found to be acceptably small—no larger than a VFI value of +/–2.5%. The goal of this projection is to illustrate the patient's possible future course, assuming that present trends continue and are not altered, for instance, by a change in therapy. Thus, the intent is not to predict what *will* happen, but rather to indicate what *could* happen if present trends were allowed to continue. Indeed, our hope is that such projections will help inform appropriate adjustments in therapy, when needed, in order to achieve less risky rates of progression in the future, and oftentimes such forward projections are quite accurate.[79] GPA projections never exceed 5 years, and are never longer than the measured follow-up period. A vertical bar to the right of the regression analysis indicates the patient's current and projected vision status.

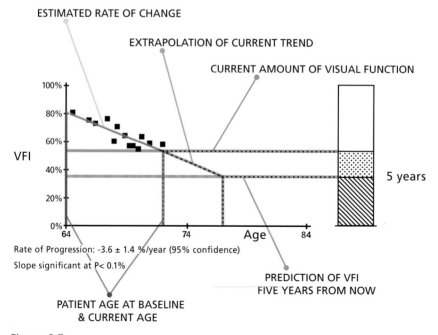

Figure 6-7

The VFI graph provides critical glaucoma management information: the rate of field progression, remaining visual field, patient age and an extrapolation of the current VFI trend.

The original HFA estimated rate of progression using linear regression analysis of Mean Deviation (MD) over time, and that analysis still is available for those preferring this approach. However, the high prevalence of developing cataract among glaucoma patients often complicates the use of MD.[80] Rate of progression estimates based on VFI have been evaluated in comparison with MD in glaucoma patients suffering from increasing cataract, in glaucoma patients free of cataract, and in glaucoma patients who have had cataract surgery during the course of follow-up. VFI based progression rates were less affected by cataract and cataract surgery than rates based on MD, but the two indices produced very similar rates in eyes that were free from cataract (Fig 6-8).[60, 81] An important difference between VFI and MD is that the MD value associated with blind fields depends upon age and testing strategy, while VFI in a blind field always is 0%, regardless of age or strategy (Fig 6-9).

Practical Clinical Use of GPA Reports

GPA analyses are available in four different report formats, ranging from a multi-page review of the patient's entire visual field history to an abbreviated summary that appears as a small part of the HFA's Single Field Analysis report. The authors recommend the GPA Summary Report as the standard printout for glaucoma management. The more detailed Full GPA Report is useful when a complete review of a patient's visual field history is needed, for instance during a presurgical review or when considering a change in baseline.

Visual Field Progression in Other Diseases

Evaluation of visual field progression in diseases other than glaucoma may require a different approach from that described above. Specifically, GPA's Pattern Deviation Change Probability significance limits are based upon empirically observed reproducibility in glaucoma patients, and thus are applicable only to that disease. Nevertheless, evaluation of series of visual fields for nonglaucomatous progression may be performed using regression analysis of VFI or Mean Deviation, and also by qualitative evaluation of the visual field series in the Overview report as described below. Diseases of interest may include retinopathies, nonglaucomatous optic neuropathies, and neurological disease (see Chapters 10 and 11).

Detection of true progression in diseases other than glaucoma can be complicated by increased testing variability associated with the disease itself. Wall et al. reported that some patients with optic neuritis demonstrated variations in visual field sensitivity that were outside the entire range of variability for normal controls. The most dramatic fluctuations occurred in a patient whose visual fields varied from normal to a hemianopic defect from one week to another and from a partial quadrant loss to a hemianopic defect at different times on the same day.[82]

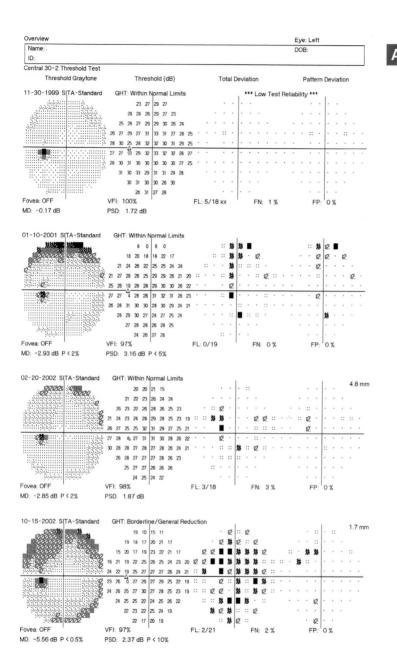

Figure 6-8

A comparison of the VFI and MD indices in cataract eyes. In this glaucoma suspect, Overview reports (A–B) show a general increase in Total Deviation loss that is typical of developing cataract. The cataract was removed in 2006, and the 2007 Total Deviation map again looks similar to the Pattern Deviation map. Since MD is a weighted average of Total Deviation, MD change closely tracked Total Deviation (C), while the VFI was as expected: considerably less affected both by the cataract and by cataract surgery (D).

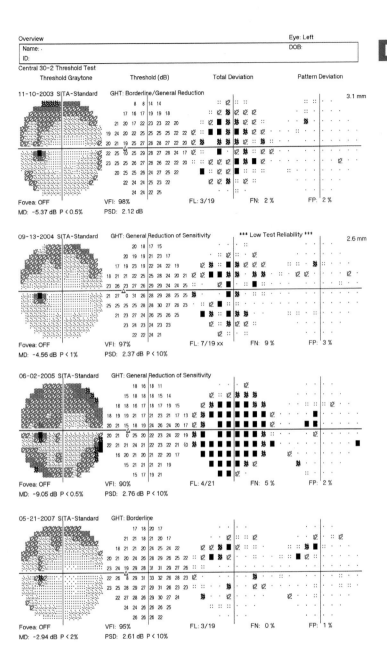

Figure 6-8

continued on the following page

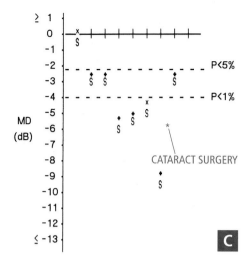

MD Slope: -0.57 ± 0.91 dB/year (95% confidence)
MD slope not significant

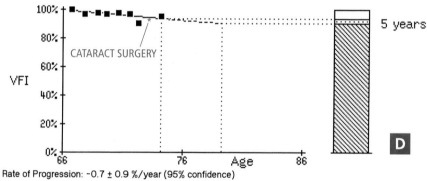

Rate of Progression: -0.7 ± 0.9 %/year (95% confidence)
Slope not significant

Figure 6-8
continued

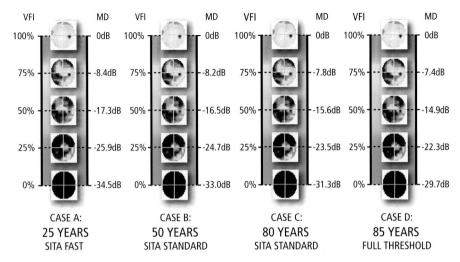

VFI		MD	VFI		MD	VFI		MD	VFI		MD
100%		0dB	100%		0dB	100%		0dB	100%		0dB
75%		-8.4dB	75%		-8.2dB	75%		-7.8dB	75%		-7.4dB
50%		-17.3dB	50%		-16.5dB	50%		-15.6dB	50%		-14.9dB
25%		-25.9dB	25%		-24.7dB	25%		-23.5dB	25%		-22.3dB
0%		-34.5dB	0%		-33.0dB	0%		-31.3dB	0%		-29.7dB

CASE A:	CASE B:	CASE C:	CASE D:
25 YEARS	50 YEARS	80 YEARS	85 YEARS
SITA FAST	SITA STANDARD	SITA STANDARD	FULL THRESHOLD

Figure 6-9
MD values associated with blind fields depend upon age and testing strategy, while VFI in a blind field is always 0%.

Alternative Analyses

OVERVIEW

The Overview report puts all of a patient's visual field tests into a single report. The Overview also is the preferred standard format in follow-up of disease other than glaucoma, such as neurological field loss (Figs 6-10 and 10-5). While this report does not quantify change, it provides a broad qualitative overview of a patient's visual field history. The Overview report also may allow you to detect and perhaps disregard tests that clearly are not representative of the patient's status, for instance because of obvious testing mistakes.

CHANGE ANALYSIS

The Change Analysis report was first offered in the original HFA over 25 years ago and has largely been replaced by the newer GPA report. However, it does contain a linear regression analysis of Mean Deviation that may be useful in certain situations. This report is fully described in the HFA Users' Manual.

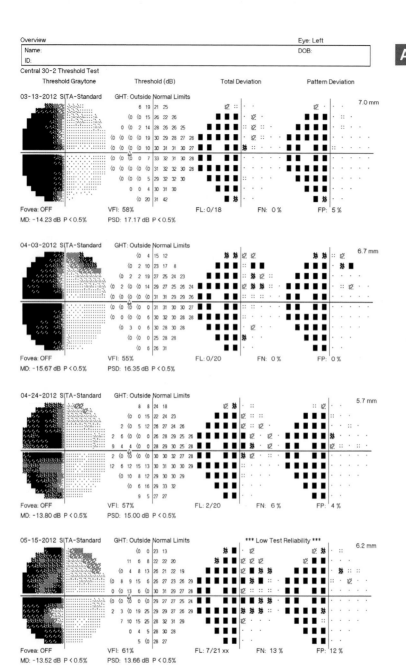

Figure 6-10

The Overview report is helpful for displaying the development of field defects over time, particularly in patients with diseases other than glaucoma. These field tests (A–B) were obtained in a young man with a very large suprasellar prolactinoma. The patient was initially treated medically with cabergoline to reduce the size of the tumor before surgery. There was a clear improvement of the visual field over the displayed 2-month period, particularly in the right eye.

Central 30-2 Threshold Test

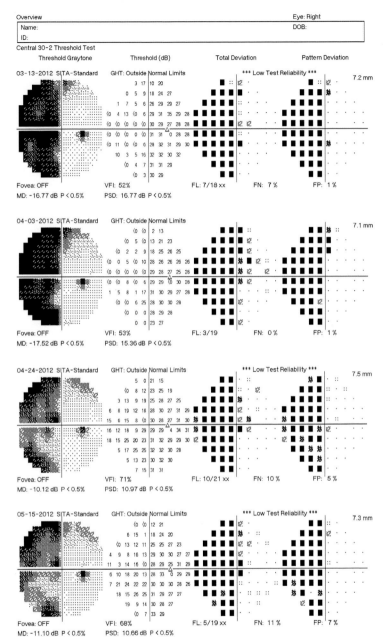

	Threshold Graytone	Threshold (dB)	Total Deviation	Pattern Deviation

03-13-2012 SITA-Standard   GHT: Outside Normal Limits   *** Low Test Reliability ***   7.2 mm

Fovea: OFF   VFI: 52%   FL: 7/18 xx   FN: 7 %   FP: 1 %
MD: -16.77 dB P < 0.5%   PSD: 16.77 dB P < 0.5%

04-03-2012 SITA-Standard   GHT: Outside Normal Limits   7.1 mm

Fovea: OFF   VFI: 53%   FL: 3/19   FN: 0 %   FP: 1 %
MD: -17.52 dB P < 0.5%   PSD: 15.36 dB P < 0.5%

04-24-2012 SITA-Standard   GHT: Outside Normal Limits   *** Low Test Reliability ***   7.5 mm

Fovea: OFF   VFI: 71%   FL: 10/21 xx   FN: 10 %   FP: 5 %
MD: -10.12 dB P < 0.5%   PSD: 10.97 dB P < 0.5%

05-15-2012 SITA-Standard   GHT: Outside Normal Limits   *** Low Test Reliability ***   7.3 mm

Fovea: OFF   VFI: 68%   FL: 5/19 xx   FN: 11 %   FP: 7 %
MD: -11.10 dB P < 0.5%   PSD: 10.66 dB P < 0.5%

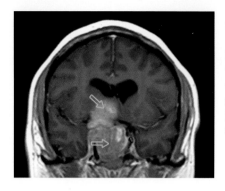

Figure 6-10 **continued**

The MRI scan (C) obtained at diagnosis shows a very large mainly suprasellar tumor measuring 4 x 4 x 7 cm with a sellar (inferior arrow) as well as large suprasellar portion (superior arrow). Tumor size diminished on cabergoline treatment.

7

Glaucomatous Visual Field Loss

G LAUCOMATOUS FIELD LOSS IS the result of axonal damage at the level of the optic disc, and is therefore the functional correlate of neural loss or reduced neural function.

Retinal Nerve Fiber Layer and Optic Disc Anatomy

Retinal ganglion cell axons follow an arcuate path to the optic nerve (Fig 7-1). Axons extending from the optic disc toward the temporal retina curve around the macular area. Neurons from the temporal superior and inferior retinal areas do not mix, but generally respect the temporal raphe. Axons also generally maintain a retinotopic organization in the optic disc in the sense that longer axons tend to be situated in the optic disc periphery, while shorter axons from ganglion cells nearer to the optic disc follow a more central course through the optic disc (Fig 7-2).

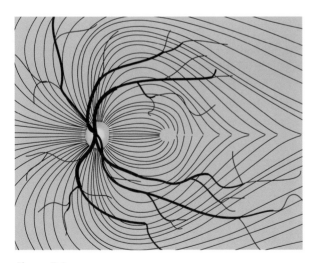

Figure 7-1
Retinal nerve fiber pattern of the central retina. Temporal nerve fibers arch around the macula and meet at the temporal raphe.

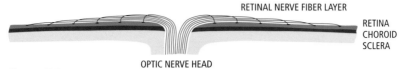

RETINAL NERVE FIBER LAYER

RETINA
CHOROID
SCLERA

OPTIC NERVE HEAD

Figure 7-2

All axons of the optic nerve converge on and exit the eye through the optic disc. Axons are systematically layered so that longer ones originating far from the disc are situated deeper in the retina and more peripherally in the optic disc .

Common Glaucomatous Field Defects and their Anatomical Correlates

Common glaucomatous visual field defects include arcuate scotomas, paracentral scotomas, and nasal steps. Mixtures of defect types often occur in the same field.

ARCUATE DEFECTS: THE BJERRUM SCOTOMA

A deep focal notch at the optic disc will lead to loss of retinal nerve fibers in the area corresponding to the notch and, therefore, to an arcuate field defect often connecting to the blind spot (see Fig 8-2A). Classically, visual field loss courses around the point of fixation and ends abruptly at the horizontal meridian corresponding to the temporal raphe, to produce what is called a Bjerrum defect.

PARACENTRAL SCOTOMAS

If the notch is partial, that is, involving only a portion of the axons in the involved area of the optic disc, it is likely that involved fibers will be of approximately equal length and originate from only a part of the arcuate segment. The resulting visual field defect is called a paracentral scotoma. Paracentral scotomas can occur any-where in the central visual field, but they are particularly common in the nasal field (Figs 7-3, 7-4).

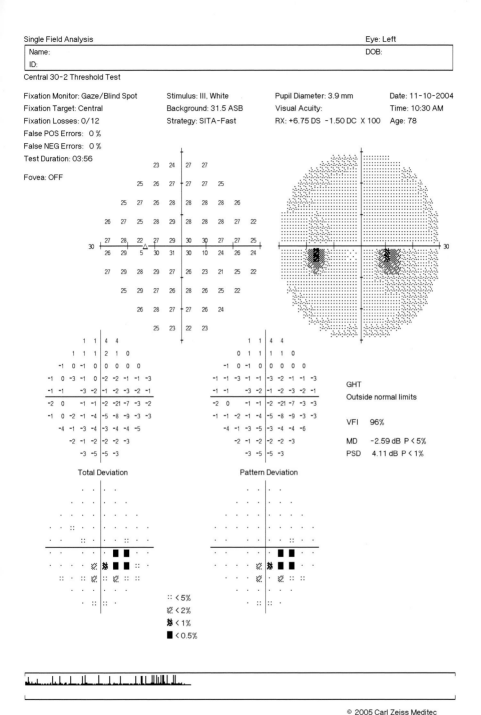

Single Field Analysis   Eye: Left

| Name: | DOB: |
| ID: | |

Central 30-2 Threshold Test

Fixation Monitor: Gaze/Blind Spot   Stimulus: III, White   Pupil Diameter: 3.9 mm   Date: 11-10-2004
Fixation Target: Central   Background: 31.5 ASB   Visual Acuity: Time: 10:30 AM
Fixation Losses: 0/12   Strategy: SITA-Fast   RX: +6.75 DS -1.50 DC X 100   Age: 78
False POS Errors: 0 %
False NEG Errors: 0 %
Test Duration: 03:56

Fovea: OFF

```
              23  24   27  27
          25  26  27   27  27  25
      25  27  26  28   28  28  28  26
   26  27  25  28  29   28  28  28  27  22
   27  28  22  27  29  30  30  27  27  25
   26  29   5  30  31  30  10  24  26  24
   27  29  28  29  27   26  23  21  25  22
      25  29  27  26   28  26  25  22
          26  28  27   27  26  24
              25  23   22  23
```

```
Total Deviation                          Pattern Deviation
        1  1   4  4                              1  1   4  4
      1  1  1  2  1  0                          0  1  1  1  1  0
   -1  0 -1  0  0  0  0  0                    -1  0  1  0  0  0  0  0
 -1  0 -3 -1  0 -2 -2 -1 -1 -3              -1 -1 -3 -1 -1 -3 -2 -1 -1 -3
 -1 -1      -3 -2 -1 -2 -3 -2 -1            -1 -1      -3 -2 -1 -2 -3 -2 -1
 -2  0      -1 -1 -2 -21 -7 -3 -2           -2  0      -1 -1 -2 -21 -7 -3 -3
 -1  0 -2 -1 -4 -5 -8 -9 -3 -3             -1 -1 -2 -1 -4 -5 -8 -9 -3 -3
   -4 -1 -3 -4 -3 -4 -4 -5                   -4 -1 -3 -5 -3 -4 -4 -6
      -2 -1 -2 -2 -2 -3                         -2 -1 -2 -2 -2 -3
         -3 -5 -5 -3                              -3 -5 -5 -3
```

GHT
Outside normal limits

VFI   96%

MD   -2.59 dB P < 5%
PSD   4.11 dB P < 1%

Total Deviation   Pattern Deviation

:: < 5%
▨ < 2%
▩ < 1%
■ < 0.5%

Figure 7-3
Glaucomatous paracentral scotoma. The expected corresponding nerve fiber layer damage is illustrated in Fig 7-4.

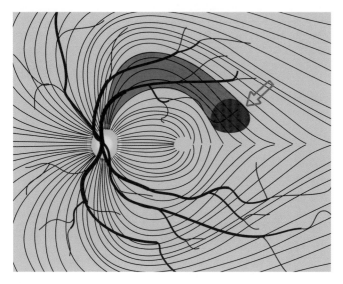

Figure 7-4

Retinal nerve fiber layer appearance in focal optic disc damage. Damaged fibers project in an arcuate pattern and are of similar length. The corresponding ganglion cells are located in the dark oval area above the temporal raphe. This illustration is intended to approximate the pattern of nerve fiber loss that would be expected to be associated with the field in Fig 7-3.

NASAL STEPS

A more widespread involvement of fibers in all parts of the optic disc will seldom be entirely symmetrical, but instead is likely to involve a larger percentage of lost fibers in either the inferior or the superior half of the optic disc. As a result, light sensitivity in the superior hemifield often will not be the same as in the lower hemifield. This frequently manifests itself as a difference in threshold sensitivity across the nasal horizontal meridian in the visual field—a nasal step (Fig 7-5).

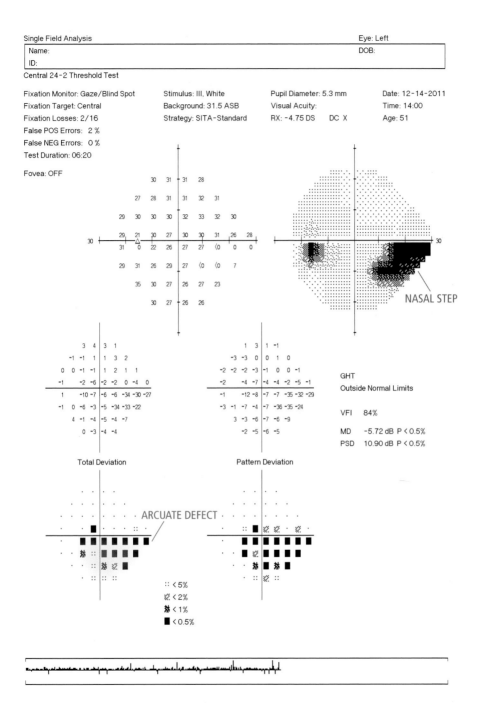

Single Field Analysis   Eye: Left

Name: DOB:

ID:

Central 24-2 Threshold Test

Fixation Monitor: Gaze/Blind Spot   Stimulus: III, White   Pupil Diameter: 5.3 mm   Date: 12-14-2011
Fixation Target: Central   Background: 31.5 ASB   Visual Acuity: Time: 14:00
Fixation Losses: 2/16   Strategy: SITA-Standard   RX: -4.75 DS   DC X   Age: 51
False POS Errors: 2 %
False NEG Errors: 0 %
Test Duration: 06:20

Fovea: OFF

GHT
Outside Normal Limits

VFI   84%

MD   -5.72 dB P < 0.5%
PSD   10.90 dB P < 0.5%

NASAL STEP

Total Deviation   Pattern Deviation

ARCUATE DEFECT

:: < 5%
🞕 < 2%
🞖 < 1%
■ < 0.5%

Figure 7-5

The grayscale map suggests a nasal step with very large sensitivity differences across the nasal horizontal meridian. However, the probability maps reveal not only a nasal step but also an arcuate defect that extends all the way to the blind spot.

Characteristics of Glaucomatous Field Loss

LOCALIZED AND GENERALIZED VISUAL FIELD LOSS

Paracentral and arcuate scotomas and nasal defects are examples of localized field loss, that is, defects that have shape. Generalized visual field loss, in contrast, is a homogeneous loss of sensitivity across the whole visual field, resulting in a depression of the hill of vision without any significant change of its shape (Fig 7-6). Homogenous visual field loss frequently is associated with cataract, especially in the age groups most at risk for glaucoma (Fig 7-7). Thus, when visual field loss is

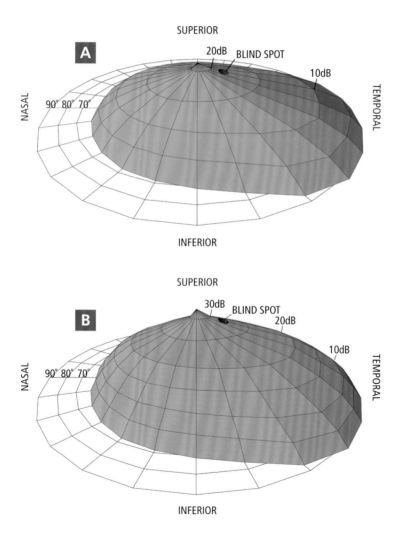

Figure 7-6
Generalized depression of the hill of vision (A) as compared to the normal hill of vision (B).

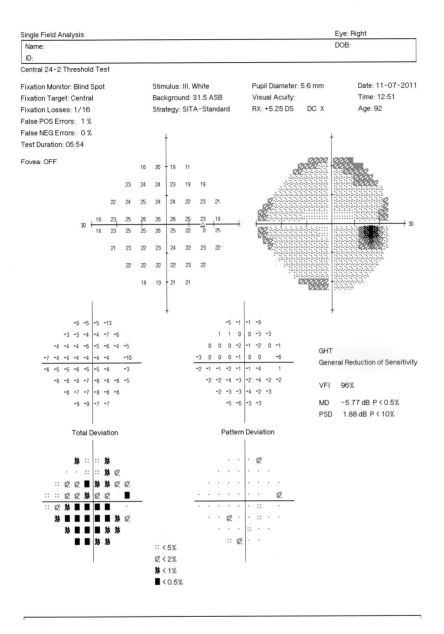

Single Field Analysis   Eye: Right

Name: DOB:

ID:

Central 24-2 Threshold Test

Fixation Monitor: Blind Spot   Stimulus: III, White   Pupil Diameter: 5.6 mm   Date: 11-07-2011
Fixation Target: Central   Background: 31.5 ASB   Visual Acuity: Time: 12:51
Fixation Losses: 1/16   Strategy: SITA-Standard   RX: +5.25 DS   DC X   Age: 92
False POS Errors: 1 %
False NEG Errors: 0 %
Test Duration: 05:54

Fovea: OFF

Total Deviation   Pattern Deviation

GHT
General Reduction of Sensitivity

VFI   96%

MD   -5.77 dB P < 0.5%
PSD   1.88 dB P < 10%

:: < 5%
✘ < 2%
✘ < 1%
■ < 0.5%

Figure 7-7

A typical cataract pattern in a 92-year-old woman with ocular hypertension and best corrected visual acuity of 0.3 (20/60). Total Deviation values are considerably more negative than Pattern Deviation values and many more test points are significantly depressed in the Total Deviation probability maps than in the Pattern Deviation probability maps. The GHT classification also is typical of cataract: General Reduction of Sensitivity. VFI is 96% while MD is significantly depressed.

encountered in test results, separating localized from generalized loss and concentrating on the former will facilitate detection of specific localized glaucomatous field damage. The Pattern Deviation maps available on the HFA STATPAC printouts are designed to do just that (see Chapter 5) (Fig 7-8).

EARLY GLAUCOMATOUS FIELD LOSS

Early glaucomatous field loss may develop very gradually over a period of several years. Local depressions of sensitivity often will come and go for quite some time before finally resolving into stable and repeatable defects.[83, 84] The Pattern Deviation maps often will expose early functional loss before it is visible in grayscale representations.

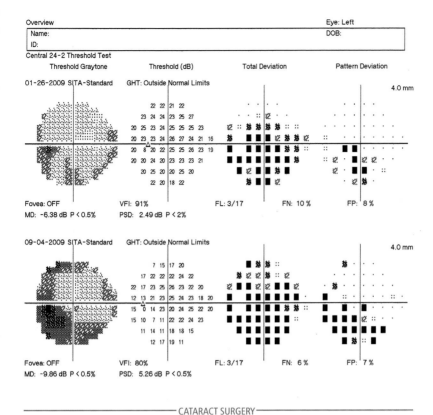

Name: DOB:
ID:

Central 24-2 Threshold Test

Threshold Graytone	Threshold (dB)	Total Deviation	Pattern Deviation

01-26-2009 SITA-Standard   GHT: Outside Normal Limits   4.0 mm

Fovea: OFF   VFI: 91%   FL: 3/17   FN: 10 %   FP: 8 %
MD: -6.38 dB P < 0.5%   PSD: 2.49 dB P < 2%

09-04-2009 SITA-Standard   GHT: Outside Normal Limits   4.0 mm

Fovea: OFF   VFI: 80%   FL: 3/17   FN: 6 %   FP: 7 %
MD: -9.86 dB P < 0.5%   PSD: 5.26 dB P < 0.5%

───────────── CATARACT SURGERY ─────────────

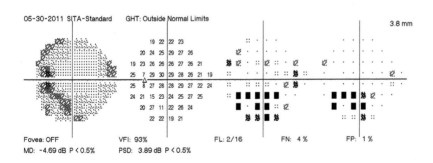

05-30-2011 SITA-Standard   GHT: Outside Normal Limits   3.8 mm

Fovea: OFF   VFI: 93%   FL: 2/16   FN: 4 %   FP: 1 %
MD: -4.69 dB P < 0.5%   PSD: 3.89 dB P < 0.5%

:: < 5%
⊠ < 2%
◈ < 1%
■ < 0.5%

Figure 7-8

Glaucoma and increasing cataract in the same eye. In the field from 2011 the cataract has been removed and the Total and Pattern Deviation probability maps are similar.

8

The Role of Perimetry in Glaucoma Management

THE GOAL OF GLAUCOMA management is to prevent loss of visual function, especially as it relates to quality of life (QOL).[71, 85] Severe glaucomatous visual field damage is associated with profound loss of QOL, and even moderate visual field loss can have significant implications[86-95] (Fig 8-1). On the other hand, therapy can have significant side effects, and maximal therapy is considerably more risky than minimal therapy. Effective diagnostic information therefore is needed in order to choose the right therapy for each patient, and in order to know when therapeutic adjustments are necessary.

Perimetry remains central to glaucoma management, not only because visual field loss is a firm diagnostic sign of glaucomatous damage, but even more importantly because knowledge of the level of and rate of vision loss provides information that is essential for the proper titration of each patient's therapy.

In the last decade we have seen the welcome arrival of increasingly effective automated ophthalmic imaging devices, and these new devices are now providing important information that is relevant to glaucoma management. However, imagers have not been shown to be as sensitive as automated perimetry to glaucomatous

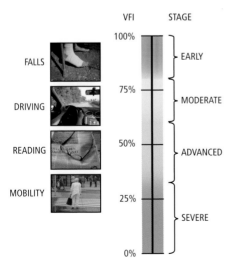

Figure 8-1

Glaucomatous field loss, particularly in the better eye, is certainly associated with quality of life. While different functions may become more obviously involved at different levels of loss, there is growing evidence that even early field loss may have more significant effects than previously thought.

progression, and cannot give us direct measurements of how well a patient is seeing.[96] Imaging studies therefore should be seen as complementary to automated perimetry and not as a replacement for measurements of visual function.[97, 98]

In this chapter we will discuss effective use of perimetry in glaucoma care. The principles are simple and straight-forward. The interpretation tools provided with the perimeter are of great help, and users can improve the effectiveness of glaucoma management by taking advantage of these methods.

Diagnosis

Glaucoma often is detected at such an advanced stage that the diagnosis is absolutely clear at the first visit.[99] A confirmatory second field test is of course not needed to make a diagnosis of glaucoma with great certainty in such situations (Fig 8-2). Often it is quite possible to diagnose glaucoma just by inspecting the optic nerve. However, qualitative optic nerve evaluation can be less reliable in many eyes, especially those having large or small optic discs (Fig 8-3).

When following patients having a normal field and elevated intraocular pressures, the situation is entirely different. In such suspects, it may take years before the first signs of field loss have appeared. With such early signs of beginning field loss, repeated perimetry is needed before an eye is considered to have glaucomatous damage.[84]

When visual field changes do appear in glaucoma suspects, the amount of confirmation required for diagnosis depends upon how suspicious we already were. In patients where suspicion is low, we may require clearly repeatable visual field loss, or the development of confirmatory structural changes. On the other hand, we might be quite quick to treat an eye showing only a suspicion of developing field loss in a patient in whom we already are treating glaucoma in the other eye or when the intraocular pressure (IOP) is quite high.

In the Ocular Hypertensive Treatment Study (OHTS) 1% to 2% per year of patients having ocular hypertension developed clear signs of glaucoma[100]—fewer than the approximately 5% diagnostic false positive rates associated both with single visual field tests and with single automated imaging analyses. In patients followed over time with a suspicion of glaucoma, an isolated Glaucoma Hemifield Test Outside Normal Limits classification or a small cluster of grey symbols in the probability maps, therefore, should not be regarded as definite proof of glaucomatous visual field damage. If, on the other hand, small clusters of defective points can be seen in

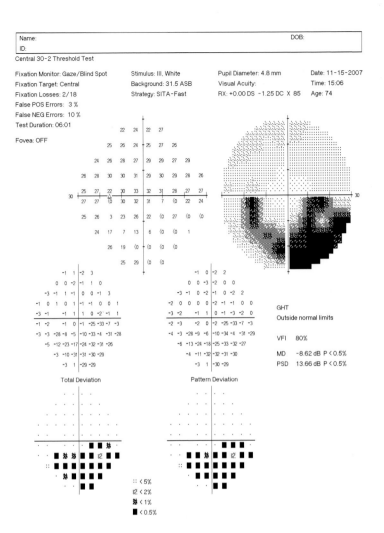

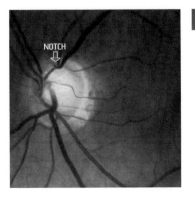

Figure 8-2

Often glaucoma is first diagnosed in patients who already have very clear disease. Diagnosis usually is easy in such cases, and there is no need to perform a confirmatory second field test to be sure of the meaning of the results. As a rule the optic disc topography also confirms obvious glaucoma. In this example, an arcuate visual field defect, also known as a Bjerrum scotoma in the lower hemifield (A), is confirmed by an optic disc notch at the opposite, superior pole of the optic disc (arrow) (B), leaving little doubt as to the diagnosis.

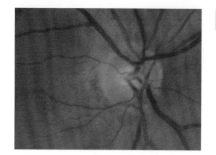

A

Figure 8-3

Glaucoma can often be diagnosed simply by inspecting the optic disc alone, but mistakes are common. Here are two examples from eyes with manifest glaucoma with field loss. These discs were shown to a large numbers of ophthalmologists in a research project undertaken in conjunction with a glaucoma conference,[134] and were misclassified by a majority of ophthalmologists. The disc in (A) was misclassified by 66% of participating doctors and the one in (C) by 53%. The field from the eye depicted in A is shown in (B), and the field corresponding to disc (C) is shown in figure (D).

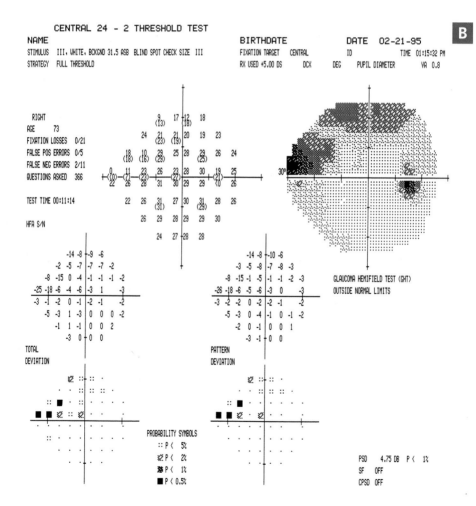

CENTRAL 24 - 2 THRESHOLD TEST

B

NAME   BIRTHDATE   DATE   02-21-95

STIMULUS   III, WHITE, BCKGND 31.5 ASB   BLIND SPOT CHECK SIZE III   FIXATION TARGET   CENTRAL   ID   TIME 01:15:32 PM

STRATEGY   FULL THRESHOLD   RX USED +5.00 DS   DCX   DEG   PUPIL DIAMETER   VA 0.8

```
RIGHT
AGE        73
FIXATION LOSSES    0/21
FALSE POS ERRORS   0/5
FALSE NEG ERRORS   2/11
QUESTIONS ASKED    366

TEST TIME 00:11:14

HFA S/N
```

```
                9   17  12   18
               (13)     (18)
          24    21   21  20   19   23
               (23) (19)
        18   19   28   25  28   29   26   24
       (18) (16) (28)             (25)
    0    11   23   26   23  28   30   19   25
   (10)  (2) (28)             (20)
    22   26   28   31   30  29   29   26
         22   26   31   27  30   31   28   26
                   (31)         (29)
              26   29   28  29   29   30
                   24   27  28   28
```

```
         -14 -8 -9  -6
    -2  -5  -7 -7  -7  -2
 -8 -15   0 -4 -1  -1  -1 -2
-25 -18 -6 -4 -6 -3  1      -3
 -3  -1 -2  0 -2 -2  -1
 -5  -3  1 -3  0  0  0 -2
    -1  1 -1  0  0  2
       -3  0  0  0
```
TOTAL
DEVIATION

```
         -14 -8 -10 -6
    -3  -5  -8 -7  -8  -3
 -8 -15 -1 -5 -1  -1  -2 -3
-26 -18 -6 -5 -6 -3  0      -3
 -3  -2  2  0 -2 -2  -1      -2
 -5  -3  0 -4 -1  0 -1 -2
    -2  0 -1  0  0  1
       -3 -1  0  0
```
PATTERN
DEVIATION

GLAUCOMA HEMIFIELD TEST (GHT)
OUTSIDE NORMAL LIMITS

PROBABILITY SYMBOLS
```
:: P <  5%
▨ P <  2%
▩ P <  1%
■ P < 0.5%
```

PSD   4.75 DB   P < 1%
SF   OFF
CPSD   OFF

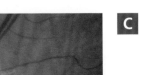

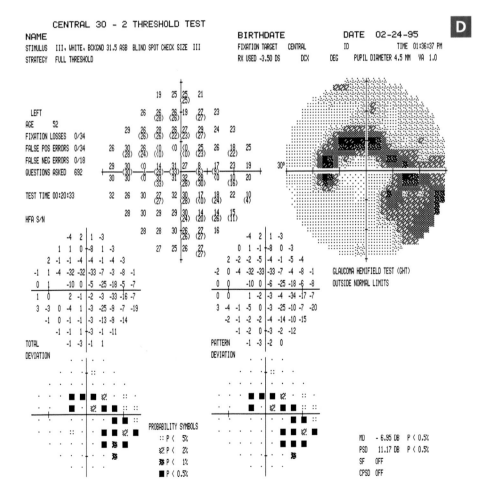

the same field area on repeated examinations, a positive diagnosis can be made with considerably increased certainty (Fig 8-4).

In glaucoma suspects and ocular hypertensive patients, it is generally not recommended to repeat questionable visual field tests during the same visit. Often, there is little urgency and in many such patients one may defer a second test until the next planned check-up.[101] On the other hand, there are other situations where it may be preferable to schedule a new test sooner. Patient age is often an important factor. Finding initial glaucomatous visual field loss in an otherwise healthy 60-year-old glaucoma suspect clearly suggests a risk of visual impairment during the patient's lifetime, while the same level of very early field loss in an 85-year-old patient may suggest low risk to future QOL.

Follow-up

In glaucoma management, the most important role of perimetry is in follow-up of patients who already have a diagnosis of glaucoma. When following glaucoma patients, the primary goal at each patient encounter must be to determine if current therapy is effective and adequate or must be changed.

CHANGING PROGRESSION PARADIGMS

The Early Manifest Glaucoma Trial demonstrated that most glaucoma eyes will show progression if followed long enough, even if treated and even if the intraocular pressure is always within the statistically normal range. In the Early Manifest Glaucoma Trial, 59% of the patients in the treated arm had shown definite progression after 8 years, and the great majority of those eyes always had IOP measurements within the normal range.[102]

Thus, we now know that progression is the rule, not the exception in glaucoma, and that fact has altered the way we react to perimetric change. We no longer automatically escalate treatment just because small but definite progression has been demonstrated. Instead, therapeutic decisions are driven by risk to QOL and commonly consider the degree of existing field loss, the rate of progression, and the patient's estimated life expectancy.

ESTABLISHING A BASELINE

Guidelines for choosing baseline tests are discussed in Chapter 6. We would only emphasize here that obtaining a representative baseline is foundational to future management decisions. Relatively few patients may require more than one or two tests to learn how to do perimetry[103–106] but additional testing of these few patients almost always is worth the extra effort.

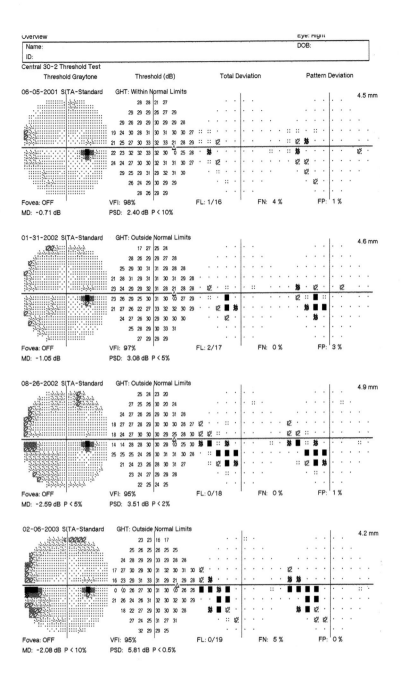

Figure 8-4

When following patients with, for instance, ocular hypertension, apparent shallow visual field defects may come and go or seemingly move around. Repeated, confirmatory findings often are needed before a diagnosis of manifest glaucoma can be made with certainty. When real field loss develops, the involved field area almost always covers an area involving several, perhaps half a dozen, test point locations.

RATES OF PROGRESSION IN GLAUCOMA

Glaucoma progression rates vary widely, even among patients under careful management, and risk factors alone cannot accurately predict which patients will progress rapidly versus slowly.[107, 108] While some patients progress very slowly and need only minimal therapy, an important minority of treated patients—perhaps one patient in six, depending upon practice type—will progress at rates that could quickly lead to disability if left unchecked (Fig 8-5).[109] In the absence of effective changes in therapy, past rates of progression have been found to be predictive of future rates.[79] Conversely, lowering IOP slows progression,[111] and progression rates have been reported to slow when pressures are lowered substantially.[112, 113] Therefore, an understanding of each patient's rate of progression is helpful in individualizing treatment and in identifying patients at high risk for progressing to visual disability.

Use of rate of progression information is now recommended in the practice guidelines of the European Glaucoma Society.[71] Elderly patients with early field defects and slow progression may not need intensified treatment, while patients of the same age having advanced field loss may require more aggressive management. Younger patients with early disease but moderate progression rates on present therapy may require early therapeutic escalation. Implicit in all this is the assumption that the goal of glaucoma therapy is to maintain each patient's visual function and related quality of life over the patient's entire lifetime. The goal might also be stated as avoidance of visual disability.

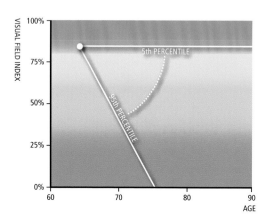

Figure 8-5

Rates of progression are highly variable in glaucoma. Here are the 5th and 95th percentile rates of progression in a large group of almost 600 glaucoma eyes under ordinary clinical care.[110]

FREQUENCY OF TESTING

European Glaucoma Society practice guidelines recommend collection of three fields per year—including baseline tests—in the first 2 years after initial diagnosis.[71] This amount of testing usually is enough to detect rapidly progressing eyes—those worsening by 2 dB/year or more.[97] The World Glaucoma Association's 2011 consensus statement on glaucoma progression makes similar suggestions,[114] and others have suggested variations on this approach.[115] In any case, ROP estimates based upon linear regression require at least five tests.

While increased testing frequency has been found to lead to earlier detection,[116] there are, of course, practical limits. Three tests per year for the first 2 years after diagnosis might be desirable, but if that cannot be done, two tests per year during the first 3 years after diagnosis is very much better than just one test per year. We must emphasize that until we have a basic assessment of rate of progression, we are basing treatment on tonometry, target pressure, and general risk factors alone. While such an approach might work for the average patient, we find that too many patients are not average.

However, it is important to understand that the frequency of field testing does not have to remain high forever. Once we have enough follow-up data to know that a patient is reasonably stable or progressing at a low and reasonably safe rate, testing intervals can be extended, perhaps to once a year. And after 6 to 8 years, if rate of progression is low or nil, it may be reasonable to extend intervals between field tests even further, as long as IOP and other clinical observations do not change.

Thus, in summary, in patients with manifest glaucoma and field loss we need to perform field testing more frequently in the first few years after diagnosis, and continue to test yearly for the next 5 years or so. Thereafter, in clearly stable patients and in elderly patients with mild visual field defects and slow rates of progression we may be able to further reduce the number of fields, in some cases perhaps to one field every second year.

In glaucoma suspects with normal fields, for instance patients with ocular hypertension, field tests are not needed nearly as often. One test per year or even every second year in some cases may be quite sufficient.

INTERPRETING VFI PROGRESSION RATES

Interpretation of rates of progression can be quite intuitive if one considers the patient's current level of visual function and life expectancy (Fig 8-6). Ideally it would be better to prevent all progression, but a minimal goal could be trying to retain at least a VFI of 50% in the better eye. The US Social Security Administration has defined an MD of -22dB as the threshold for visual disability.[44] An MD of -22dB corresponds to a VFI of approximately 30%.

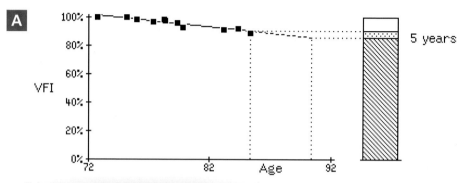

Rate of Progression: -0.9 ± 0.2 %/year (95% confidence)
Slope significant at P < 0.1%

Figure 8-6
The statistical significance of the VFI slope often is of little interest. In (A) VFI slope is statistically significant but so shallow as to pose little threat in the patient's lifetime, providing little reason to depart from current therapy. Compare this to (E, page 100) where the slope appears to be immediately threatening; here, only four fields have been taken, and the statistical slope therefore has not been calculated. In (E) particularly rapid progression in an operated eye with pressures in the upper teens is represented, and this illustrates that there sometimes may be no need to wait for a fifth field and statistical analysis of slope before taking clinical action. The slopes in (C) and (D) are also threatening and suggest that considerably more intensive treatment, perhaps a radical change of treatment, should be considered. (C) is as serious as (D), because the patient in (C) is much younger. (B) represents a common clinical situation: the progression rate does not pose an imminent threat, but progression is certainly important clinically, despite the patient's age. In such situations more intensive therapy usually should be considered and, as always, weighed against therapeutic risks and the likelihood of success.

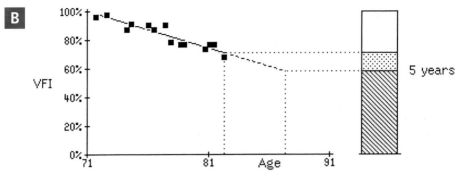

Rate of Progression: −2.5 ± 0.7 %/year (95% confidence)
Slope significant at P < 0.1%

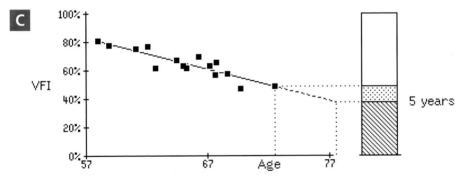

Rate of Progression: −2.2 ± 0.7 %/year (95% confidence)
Slope significant at P < 0.1%

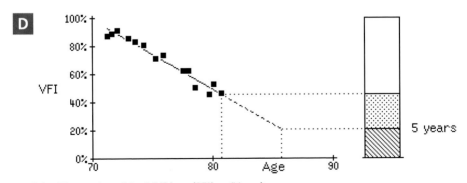

Rate of Progression: −5.0 ± 0.7 %/year (95% confidence)
Slope significant at P < 0.1%

First chosen baseline test not used in order
to correct for marked learning effects.

| Name: | DOB: |
| ID: | |

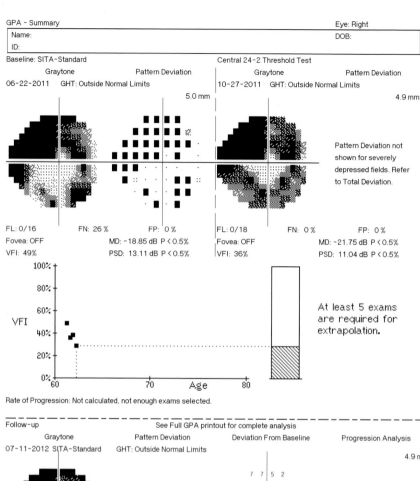

Baseline: SITA-Standard   Central 24-2 Threshold Test

Graytone   Pattern Deviation   Graytone   Pattern Deviation

06-22-2011   GHT: Outside Normal Limits   10-27-2011   GHT: Outside Normal Limits

5.0 mm   4.9 mm

Pattern Deviation not
shown for severely
depressed fields. Refer
to Total Deviation.

FL: 0/16	FN: 26 %	FP: 0 %	FL: 0/18	FN: 0 %	FP: 0 %
Fovea: OFF	MD: -18.85 dB P < 0.5%		Fovea: OFF	MD: -21.75 dB P < 0.5%	
VFI: 49%	PSD: 13.11 dB P < 0.5%		VFI: 36%	PSD: 11.04 dB P < 0.5%	

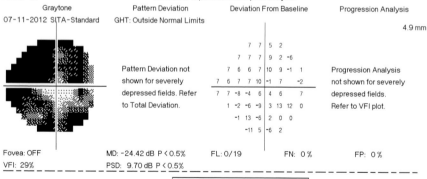

At least 5 exams
are required for
extrapolation.

Rate of Progression: Not calculated, not enough exams selected.

Follow-up   See Full GPA printout for complete analysis

Graytone   Pattern Deviation   Deviation From Baseline   Progression Analysis

07-11-2012 SITA-Standard   GHT: Outside Normal Limits

4.9 mm

Pattern Deviation not
shown for severely
depressed fields. Refer
to Total Deviation.

```
            7  7  5  2
            7  7  7  9  2 -6
      7  6  6  7 10  9 -1  1
   7  6  7  7 10 -1  7    -2
   7  7 -8 -4  6  4  6     7
   1 -2 -6 -9  3 13 12  0
     -1 13 -6  2  0  0
    -11  5 -6  2
```

Progression Analysis
not shown for severely
depressed fields.
Refer to VFI plot.

| Fovea: OFF | MD: -24.42 dB P < 0.5% | FL: 0/19 | FN: 0 % | FP: 0 % |
| VFI: 29% | PSD: 9.70 dB P < 0.5% | | | |

*** Baseline MD is out of range ***
Previous Follow-up Exams:
        02-03-2012

:: < 5%	⅄ P < 5% Deterioration
⌕ < 2%	▲ P < 5% (2 consecutive)
⚵ < 1%	▲ P < 5% (3+ consecutive)
■ < 0.5%	X Out of Range

Notes:

DATA MANAGEMENT AND NETWORKING

Proper use of progression analysis applications requires that all relevant fields be properly identified and available for analysis. Patient name, birth date, and identification number must be consistent across all visual field test results if analysis programs are to recognize the tests as all belonging to a single patient (see Fig 2-2). The best way to ensure that the identification data are consistent is to establish a disciplined protocol for entering such information at each perimetric visit. We suggest recalling each returning patient's identification data from previous tests using the Humphrey perimeter's "Recall patient data" function, or to connecting your HFAs to your Electronic Health Record system, for instance using ZEISS FORUM® software.

Clinics having multiple perimeters may have performed some of a patient's tests on one perimeter and other tests on another instrument, and must make sure that all tests are available to the progression analysis program being used. In the past, this has been achieved by manually transferring test results between perimeters using floppy discs or USB compatible thumb drives, but it is now possible to network all perimeters to a centrally maintained database containing all patient tests. All HFA perimeters built since the year 2002 are equipped with Ethernet and can be networked using ZEISS FORUM® software, so that they all can refer to a single central archive of test results. It also is worth noting that patient test results obtained or stored on older HFA1 and HFA2 instruments may be electronically transferred to newer instruments and/or to a FORUM central archive. Test results from these legacy instruments may also be used in current progression analyses.

9

Integrating Structural and Functional Measurements

AUTOMATED IMAGING AND QUANTITATIVE measurement of ocular structures have become increasingly available in clinical practice worldwide. Posterior segment metrics include optic nerve topography, retinal nerve fiber layer (RNFL) thickness, and macular ganglion cell layer thickness. Measurements of anterior segment structures are becoming increasingly available as well. With this new information has come a clear need to integrate automated imaging findings into a diagnostic picture that already includes automated perimetry, tonometry, photography, clinical examination, and patient history.

Relationship between Structural and Functional Measurements

In principle, structural and functional findings should corroborate and confirm each other if the measurements are of sufficient accuracy and precision (Figs 9-1 and 9-3). However most investigators have found that current structural metrics explain less than half of contemporary perimetric results, and vice versa.[117-122] Thus, there frequently will be cases where the perimetry is outside normal limits and the structural findings are not, and also cases where the opposite will be true[123] (Fig. 9-2). Similarly, we know that we can see significant RNFL thickness change from baseline that is not confirmed by progression analysis of the corresponding series of visual fields, and also the opposite case.

Strengths and Weaknesses

Much has been made of the fact that patients can locally lose about 30% of their retinal nerve fibers before the corresponding perimetric test point location falls outside the normal range.[124]

Less has been said about the fact that patients also can lose about a third of their average nerve fiber layer thickness and still be within normal limits for RNFL thickness. Similarly, while the future of imaging really is quite bright, current structural measurements can quantify fewer steps from normal to blind than can be determined using standard automated perimetry.[96]

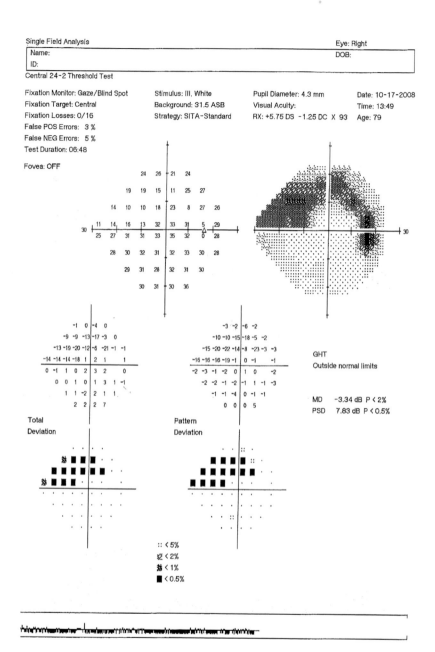

Single Field Analysis   Eye: Right

Name: DOB:

ID:

Central 24-2 Threshold Test

Fixation Monitor: Gaze/Blind Spot   Stimulus: III, White   Pupil Diameter: 4.3 mm   Date: 10-17-2008
Fixation Target: Central   Background: 31.5 ASB   Visual Acuity: Time: 13:49
Fixation Losses: 0/16   Strategy: SITA-Standard   RX: +5.75 DS -1.25 DC X 93   Age: 79
False POS Errors: 3 %
False NEG Errors: 5 %
Test Duration: 06:48

Fovea: OFF

GHT
Outside normal limits

MD   -3.34 dB P < 2%
PSD   7.83 dB P < 0.5%

Total Deviation

Pattern Deviation

:: < 5%
▨ < 2%
▩ < 1%
■ < 0.5%

Figure 9-1

Oftentimes visual function data are corroborated by structural data. The arcuate scotoma in the upper hemifield (A) is in good agreement with optical coherence tomography (OCT) findings showing thinning of the retinal nerve fiber layer (RNFL) in the inferior quadrant (B).

Name:

	OD	OS	
Exam Date:	2008-10-17	2008-10-17	CZMI
Exam Time:	14:32	14:33	
Serial Number:	4000-1350	4000-1350	
Signal Strength:	7/10	6/10	

ID:
DOB:
Gender:
Doctor:

ZEISS

ONH and RNFL OU Analysis: Optic Disc Cube 200x200   OD ● | ● OS

RNFL Thickness Map

350
175
0 µm

	OD	OS
Average RNFL Thickness	65 µm	80 µm
RNFL Symmetry	40%	
Rim Area	1,15 mm²	1,39 mm²
Disc Area	2,48 mm²	2,49 mm²
Average C/D Ratio	0,72	0,68
Vertical C/D Ratio	0,77	0,64
Cup Volume	0,246 mm³	0,192 mm³

RNFL Thickness Map

350
175
0 µm

RNFL Deviation Map

RNFL Deviation Map

Neuro-retinal Rim Thickness

µm ——— OD - - - OS

800
400
0

0 TEMP | SUP | NAS | INF | TEMP

Disc Center (-0,03,-0,03) mm
Extracted Horizontal Tomogram

Disc Center (0,21,0,06) mm
Extracted Horizontal Tomogram

RNFL Thickness

µm ——— OD - - - OS

200
100
0

0 TEMP | 30 | 60 SUP | 90 | 120 NAS | 150 | 180 INF | 210 | 240 TEMP

Extracted Vertical Tomogram

Extracted Vertical Tomogram

Diversified:
Distribution of Normals

NA   95% 5% 1%

90

S
55 T | N 63
I
53

106

S
61 N | T 54
I
100

RNFL Quadrants

RNFL Circular Tomogram

RNFL Circular Tomogram

RNFL Clock Hours

97
86   88
60   76
49   54
57   59
49   62
   47

130
98   88
72   58
54   41
56   62
74   125
  101

SW Ver: 6.0.0.599
Copyright 2011
Carl Zeiss Meditec, Inc
All Rights Reserved
Page 1 of 1

Comments

Doctor's Signature

Analysis Edited: 2008-10-17 14:34

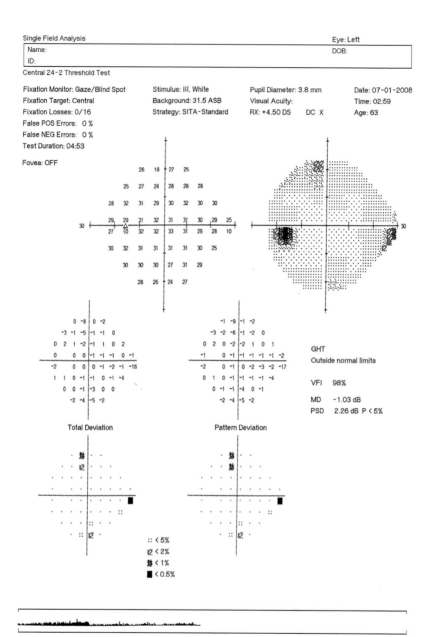

Figure 9-2

This subject was randomly recruited to participate in a population-based clinical trial, and in this situation, the visual field findings (A) are difficult to interpret. While the GHT is outside normal limits, the pattern of loss shown on the probability maps is not as compelling as it might be if seen in a glaucoma suspect. The OCT findings (B) in this eye all are within normal limits, however; taking both function and structure into account, we judged the suspicion of glaucoma to be low.

Name:		**OD**	**OS**	
ID:	Exam Date:	2008-07-01	2008-07-01	CZMI
DOB:	Exam Time:	11:23	11:25	
Gender:	Serial Number:	4000-1350	4000-1350	
Doctor:	Signal Strength:	10/10	9/10	

ONH and RNFL OU Analysis: Optic Disc Cube 200x200   OD ● ● OS

RNFL Thickness Map

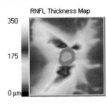

	OD	**OS**
Average RNFL Thickness	97 µm	98 µm
RNFL Symmetry	80%	
Rim Area	1,02 mm²	1,16 mm²
Disc Area	1,51 mm²	1,64 mm²
Average C/D Ratio	0,57	0,54
Vertical C/D Ratio	0,54	0,49
Cup Volume	0,156 mm³	0,144 mm³

RNFL Thickness Map

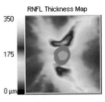

RNFL Deviation Map

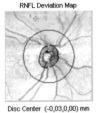

Disc Center (-0,03,0,00) mm
Extracted Horizontal Tomogram

Extracted Vertical Tomogram

RNFL Circular Tomogram

Neuro-retinal Rim Thickness

µm   — OD --- OS

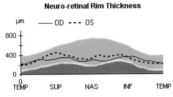

```
800
400
0
   0   SUP   NAS   INF   TEMP
  TEMP
```

RNFL Thickness

µm   — OD --- OS

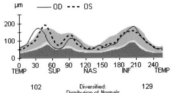

```
200
100
0
   0   30  60  90  120 150 180 210 240
  TEMP   SUP      NAS      INF   TEMP
```

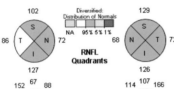

Diversified:
Distribution of Normals

       102   129
        ┌─S─┐   ┌─S─┐
   86 T │ N 72   68 N │ T 72
        └─I─┘   └─I─┘
       127   126

NA   95% 5% 1%

RNFL Quadrants

```
      67  88                  107 166
   152      95          114        85
121                  83
  59      54          57        52
   77   67              63    77
   149 148 84            93 147 137
```

RNFL Clock Hours

RNFL Deviation Map

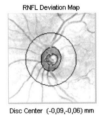

Disc Center (-0,09,-0,06) mm
Extracted Horizontal Tomogram

Extracted Vertical Tomogram

RNFL Circular Tomogram

Comments	Doctor's Signature	
		SW Ver: 6.0.0.599
Analysis Edited: 2008-07-01 11:25		Copyright 2011 Carl Zeiss Meditec, Inc All Rights Reserved Page 1 of 1

We make these observations simply to point out 1) that there is ample room for further development of all of our diagnostics, 2) that automated perimetry continues to occupy an important and central role in the management of ophthalmic disease, and 3) that integration of structural and function findings remains an inexact but highly promising opportunity.

Practical Considerations

In evaluating diagnostic findings that are outside normal limits, it may be helpful to think a little about the interplay between the diagnostic specificity and disease likelihood in a clinical population. For instance, the Humphrey perimeter's Glaucoma Hemifield Test (GHT) was designed to have an overall specificity of approximately 94% and thus must be expected to produce about 6% false positive findings in normal subjects. Similarly, most structural metrics are designed to fall outside normal limits in 5% of normals, even under ideal circumstances.

GHT findings that are outside normal limits in a subject randomly chosen from a population having 1% prevalence of glaucoma thus would be 6 times more likely to be a false positive diagnostic finding than to be associated with true disease. In contrast, a positive GHT finding in a referral practice where 50% of newly referred patients typically do have glaucoma would be about 13 times more likely to be associated with true glaucoma than a false positive finding.

Therefore, in patients in whom we have a low level of suspicion, it may be prudent to require both structural and functional change, while in high-risk populations it might be sufficient for findings to be outside normal limits in either structure or function. In all cases, it is crucial to adjust clinical interpretation of diagnostic findings on the basis of the level of suspicion we had before the test was done—a factor called the pretest probability of disease.

General Guidelines

HIGH-RISK PATIENTS

Positive findings in either structure or function may be sufficient to merit a diagnosis of glaucoma. For example, a patient having a normal field but very high pressures and a clearly glaucomatous disc may well merit a diagnosis of glaucoma.

LOW-RISK PATIENTS

Low-risk patients may require significant corroboration of diagnostic findings. Ideally, both structure and function must be outside normal limits, but corroboration from other data sources may replace one or the other. For example, an outside normal limits visual field result in a patient having a positive family history for glaucoma but a normal looking disc and a normal intraocular pressure probably requires additional corroborating evidence of glaucoma. Such corroborating evidence might come at a later time, during routine follow-up.

Looking Toward the Future

Currently, we have the ability to present structural and functional findings in a single report (Fig 9-3). Clear opportunities exist to construct analyses that combine structural and functional data.[125] We can imagine a combination analysis that integrates multiple optical coherence tomography (OCT) metrics—RNFL thickness, optic nerve measurements, and ganglion cell thickness—with perimetry findings to produce a single highly specific and sensitive diagnostic analysis. Perhaps a slightly suspicious perimetry finding, combined with a similarly subtle structural finding might be so unusual in normal subjects as to confirm a diagnosis of glaucoma in a patient having only elevated pressures. The same might be done with combination analyses for progression,[126, 127] perhaps reducing the number of patient visits and the time required to identify rapidly progressing patients.

Automated ophthalmic imaging is rapidly evolving and will improve significantly in the coming years. Connectivity initiatives currently underway will provide infrastructure that will simplify the process of combining structural and functional information available into a single analysis. The future is bright.

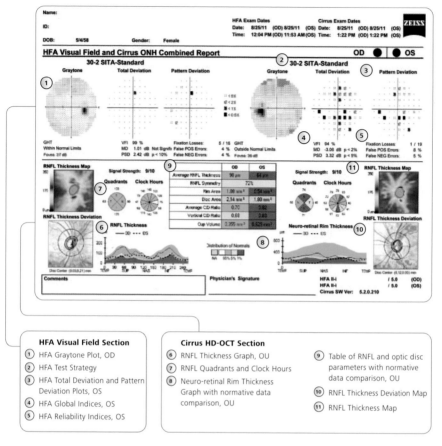

Figure 9-3

Visual field and Spectral Domain OCT findings from both eyes now can be presented in a single report using ZEISS FORUM software.

10

Neurological
Visual Field Loss

BECAUSE THE VISUAL SYSTEM occupies or passes through so much of the brain, patterns of visual field loss caused by neurological disease often are quite specific. Before the advent of neuroimaging, visual fields frequently were the best indicators of the location, and sometimes even the nature, of central nervous system disease. Even today perimetry often can provide a simple and cost-effective aid to neurological diagnosis, and neurological disease often is identified accidentally during visual field testing, such as in follow-up examination of glaucoma patients. Modern practice emphasizes testing in the central field in assessing neurological field loss.[28]

Optic Nerve Disease

Unilateral optic nerve disease naturally produces field defects in just the affected eye. A central scotoma is the typical pattern of field loss for several types of optic nerve disease, such as optic neuritis (Fig 10-1), many toxic reactions, and mechanical compression of the nerve. The size of the visual field defect varies, and reduced visual acuity often is associated with larger scotomas. If the damage is small enough that visual acuity still is normal or only slightly depressed, the scotoma may be so small that sensitivity is only marginally depressed at some central points in the standard 30-2 or 24-2 test point patterns. A 10-2 test is likely to show more in such cases. Optic neuritis can cause a large variety of both diffuse and localized visual field defects, some of which may even resemble those typical of glaucoma.[128, 129]

Anterior ischemic optic neuropathy usually results in sudden and large loss of visual function. Field loss frequently is large, with sizeable areas of absolute damage. Many different patterns are possible, with altitudinal hemianopia perhaps being the most common. Just as with other hemianopias, those in optic nerve infarction are often incomplete, and it is common to see areas of diminished function in the less affected hemifield as well.

Early phase optic disc edema typically produces only an enlargement of the blind spot, which may be surrounded by a zone of relative loss of sensitivity. However, diagnosis more often is made with ophthalmoscopy or fundus imaging and not with

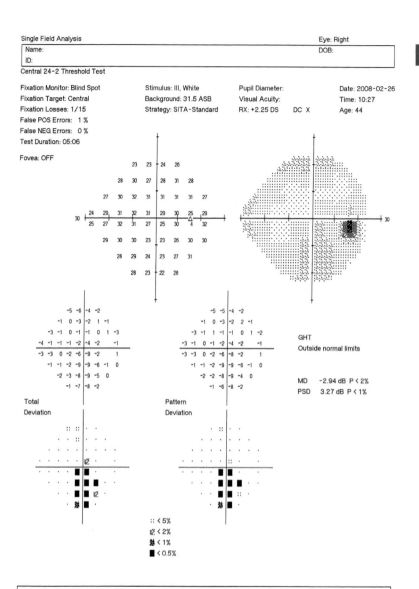

Name: DOB:

ID:

A

Central 24-2 Threshold Test

Fixation Monitor: Blind Spot   Stimulus: III, White   Pupil Diameter: Date: 2008-02-26

Fixation Target: Central   Background: 31.5 ASB   Visual Acuity: Time: 10:27

Fixation Losses: 1/15   Strategy: SITA-Standard   RX: +2.25 DS   DC X   Age: 44

False POS Errors: 1 %

False NEG Errors: 0 %

Test Duration: 05:06

Fovea: OFF

GHT

Outside normal limits

MD   -2.94 dB P < 2%

PSD   3.27 dB P < 1%

Total Deviation

Pattern Deviation

:: < 5%

< 2%

< 1%

■ < 0.5%

Figure 10-1

Visual fields from an eye with retrobulbar optic neuritis. A 45-year-old woman sought medical advice after noticing blurred central vision in her right eye. Best corrected visual acuity was 0.4 (20/50), color vision testing was deficient, and the field showed the central defects (A). One week later the eye had lost one more line of visual acuity (VA), and the central scotoma was larger and more clearly visible in the grayscale map than before (B). The patient gradually improved and one month later VA was 0.7 (20/30), but the visual field defects remained very distinct in the probability maps (C). After 3 months the patient had recovered with a normal field (D), a visual acuity of 1.0 (20/20), and normal color vision.

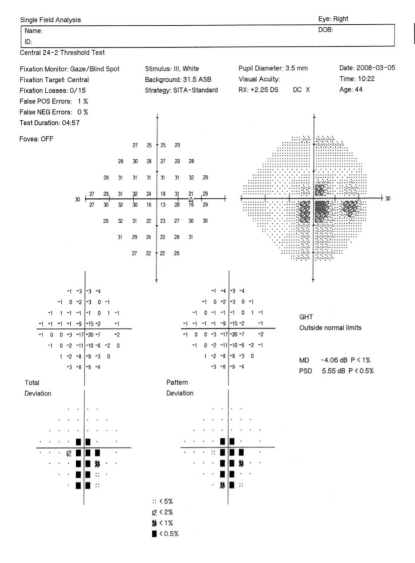

Single Field Analysis   Eye: Right

Name:	DOB:
ID:	

B

Central 24-2 Threshold Test

Fixation Monitor: Gaze/Blind Spot   Stimulus: III, White   Pupil Diameter: 3.5 mm   Date: 2008-03-05
Fixation Target: Central   Background: 31.5 ASB   Visual Acuity: Time: 10:22
Fixation Losses: 0/15   Strategy: SITA-Standard   RX: +2.25 DS   DC X   Age: 44
False POS Errors: 1 %
False NEG Errors: 0 %
Test Duration: 04:57

Fovea: OFF

```
              27  25   25  23
          28  30  28   27  29  28
      28  31  31   31   31  31  32  29
30  27  29  31   32  24  18  31  21  29
    27  30  32   30  16  13  26  16  29
      29  32  31   22  23  27  30  30
          31  29  24   22  28  31
              27  22   22  26
```

Total Deviation
```
      -1  -3 |-3  -4
  -1   0  -2 |-3   0  -1
-1   1  -1  -1 |-1   0   1  -1
-1  -1  -1  -1 |-9 -15  -2      -1
-1   0   0  -3 |-17 -20 -7      -2
  -1   0  -2 -11 |-10  -6  -2   0
    1  -2  -8 |-9  -3   0
      -3  -8 |-9  -4
```

Pattern Deviation
```
      -1  -4 |-3  -4
  -1   0  -2 |-3   0  -1
-1   0  -1  -1 |-1   0   1  -1
-1  -1  -1  -1 |-9 -15  -2      -1
-1   0   0  -3 |-17 -20 -7      -2
  -1   0  -2 -11 |-10  -6  -2  -1
    1  -2  -8 |-9  -3   0
      -3  -8 |-9  -4
```

GHT
Outside normal limits

MD   -4.06 dB P < 1%
PSD   5.55 dB P < 0.5%

Total Deviation

Pattern Deviation

```
:: < 5%
✕ < 2%
▨ < 1%
■ < 0.5%
```

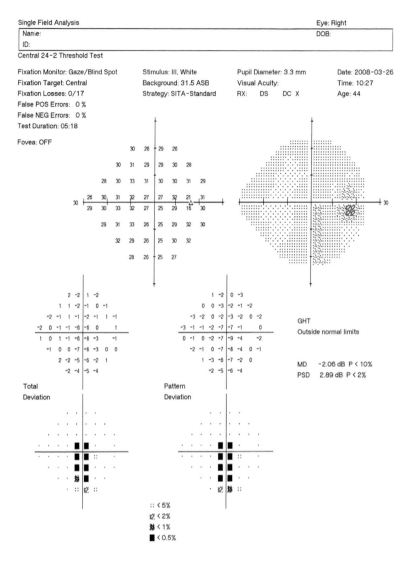

Single Field Analysis   Eye: Right

Name: DOB:
ID:

Central 24-2 Threshold Test

Fixation Monitor: Gaze/Blind Spot   Stimulus: III, White   Pupil Diameter: 3.3 mm   Date: 2008-03-26
Fixation Target: Central   Background: 31.5 ASB   Visual Acuity: Time: 10:27
Fixation Losses: 0/17   Strategy: SITA-Standard   RX: DS   DC X   Age: 44
False POS Errors: 0 %
False NEG Errors: 0 %
Test Duration: 05:18

Fovea: OFF

```
                  30  26   29  26
              30  31  29   29  30  28
          28  30  33  31   30  30  31  29
      30  26  30  31  32  27  27  32  21  31
          29  30  33  32  27  25  29  16  30
          29  31  33  26   25  29  32  30
              32  29  26   25  30  32
                  28  26   25  27
```

```
   Total                          Pattern
   Deviation                      Deviation

    2  -2  | 1  -2                   1  -2 | 0  -3
  1   1  -2 |-1   0  -1              0   0  -3 |-2  -1  -2
 -2  -1   1  -1 |-2  -1   1  -1     -3  -2   0  -2 |-3  -2   0  -2
 -2   0  -1  -1  -6 |-6   0     1   -3  -1  -1  -2  -7 |-7  -1      0
  1   0   1  -1  -6 |-8  -3      -1   0  -1   0  -2  -7 |-9  -4     -2
 -1   0   0  -7 |-8  -3   0   0    -2  -1   0  -7 |-8  -4   0  -1
    2  -2  -5 |-6  -2   1            1  -3  -6 |-7  -2   0
       -2  -4 |-5  -4                   -2  -5 |-6  -4
```

GHT
Outside normal limits

MD   -2.06 dB P < 10%
PSD   2.89 dB P < 2%

Total   Pattern
Deviation   Deviation

:: < 5%
✗ < 2%
✦ < 1%
■ < 0.5%

Name:	DOB:
ID:	

D

Central 24-2 Threshold Test

Fixation Monitor: Gaze/Blind Spot   Stimulus: III, White   Pupil Diameter: 3.9 mm   Date: 06-12-2008
Fixation Target: Central   Background: 31.5 ASB   Visual Acuity: Time: 7:32 AM
Fixation Losses: 0/14   Strategy: SITA-Standard   RX: +2.50 DS   DC X   Age: 44
False POS Errors: 1 %
False NEG Errors: 0 %
Test Duration: 04:31

Fovea: OFF

```
                25  27    27  30
            32  31  29   29  31  29
        30  32  32  31   32  32  32  29
    30  28  28  32  33   33  33  32  19  31
        30  31  33  33   33  33  32  20  29
        29  32  32  31   30  31  30  30
            31  29  29   29  30  31
                30  27    30  27
```

Total Deviation
```
        -3  -1  -1   2
     2   0  -2  -1   2   0
   1   1   1  -1   0   1   1   0
 0  -2   0   0  -1   0   0       1
 2   1   1   0   0   0   0      -2
  -1   1  -1  -2  -3  -1  -1   0
   1  -2  -2  -3  -1   0
     0  -3  -1  -4
```

Pattern Deviation
```
        -4  -2  -2   1
     1  -1  -3  -2   1  -1
   0   0   0  -2  -1   0   0  -2
-1  -3  -1  -1  -2  -1  -1       0
 1  -1   0  -1  -1  -1  -1      -3
  -2   0  -2  -3  -4  -2  -2  -2
   0  -3  -3  -4  -2  -1
    -1  -4  -2  -5
```

GHT
Within normal limits

VFI   100%

MD   -0.43 dB
PSD   1.37 dB

Total Deviation

Pattern Deviation

```
:: < 5%
⚹ < 2%
⚸ < 1%
■ < 0.5%
```

perimetry. Nevertheless, patients with optic disc edema may benefit from regular visual field testing, because longstanding optic disc edema can produce secondary progressive optic atrophy. Perimetry may show field loss in such cases (Fig 10-2). Threshold tests using the 30-2 and 24-2 patterns are suitable for following these patients.

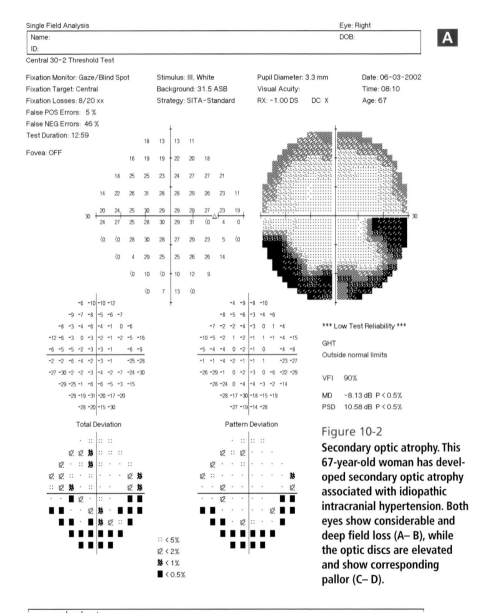

Figure 10-2

Secondary optic atrophy. This 67-year-old woman has developed secondary optic atrophy associated with idiopathic intracranial hypertension. Both eyes show considerable and deep field loss (A– B), while the optic discs are elevated and show corresponding pallor (C– D).

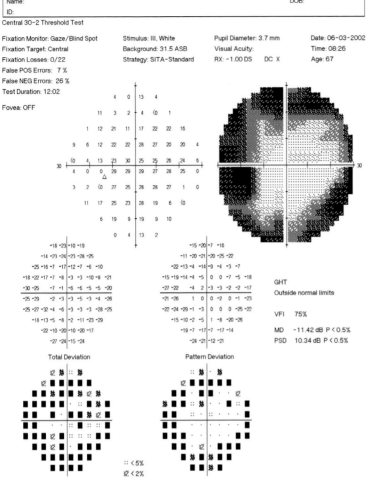

Single Field Analysis   Eye: Left

Name: DOB:
ID: **B**

Central 30-2 Threshold Test

Fixation Monitor: Gaze/Blind Spot   Stimulus: III, White   Pupil Diameter: 3.7 mm   Date: 06-03-2002
Fixation Target: Central   Background: 31.5 ASB   Visual Acuity: Time: 08:26
Fixation Losses: 0/22   Strategy: SITA-Standard   RX: -1.00 DS   DC X   Age: 67
False POS Errors: 7 %
False NEG Errors: 26 %
Test Duration: 12:02

Fovea: OFF

```
              4   0 | 13   4
          11  3   2 | 4  (0   1
       1  12  21 11 |17  22  22  16
    9  6  12  22 22 |28  27  20  20   4
30 (0  4  13  23 30 |25  25  26  24   6   30
    4  0   0  29 29 |29  27  28  25   0
       3  2  (0  27 |25  28  28  27   1   0
      11 17  25 23 |28  19   6  (0
          6  19  9 |19   9  10
              0   4 | 13   2
```

```
-18 -23 -10 -19                          -15 -20 -7 -16
-14 -24 -24 -23 -28 -25                 -11 -20 -21 -20 -25 -22
-25 -16 -7 -17 -12 -7 -6 -10            -22 -13 -4 -14 -9 -4 -3 -7
-18 -22 -17 -7 -8 -3 -3 -10 -8 -21      -15 -19 -14 -4 -5  0  0 -7 -5 -18    GHT
-30 -25 -7 -1 -6 -6 -5 -5 -20           -27 -22 -4 2 -3 -3 -2 -2 -17         Outside normal limits
-25 -29 -2 -3 -3 -5 -3 -4 -26           -21 -26  1  0 0 -2  0 -1 -23
-25 -27 -32 -4 -6 -3 -3 -3 -28 -25      -22 -24 -29 -1 -3  0  0  0 -25 -22   VFI   75%
-18 -13 -5 -8 -2 -11 -23 -29            -15 -10 -2 -5  1 -8 -20 -26
-22 -10 -20 -10 -20 -17                 -19 -7 -17 -7 -17 -14                MD   -11.42 dB  P < 0.5%
-27 -24 -15 -24                          -24 -21 -12 -21                      PSD  10.34 dB  P < 0.5%
```

Total Deviation   Pattern Deviation

:: < 5%
⚲ < 2%
✷ < 1%
■ < 0.5%

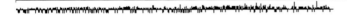

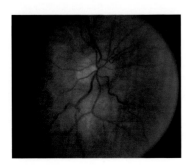   **C**   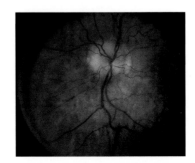   **D**

Drusen of the optic disc produce arcuate defects that may be indistinguishable from those caused by glaucoma (Fig 10-3). Associated visual field loss may be progressive.

Serious thyroid ophthalmopathy causes field defects because of optic nerve involvement. The appearance of such defects varies tremendously, but in contrast with

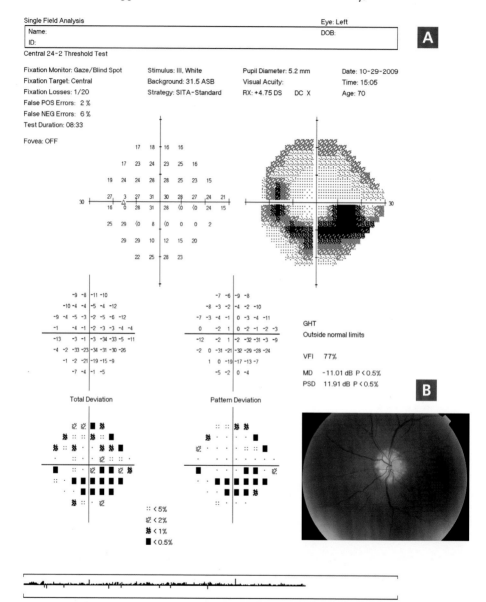

Figure 10-3
Visual fields from an eye diagnosed to have optic disc drusen (A). Drusen are often difficult to see (B), but usually become more apparent with age. Field defects frequently are slowly progressive.

glaucomatous defects, they may regress or even disappear after successful treatment of the ophthalmopathy (Fig 10-4).

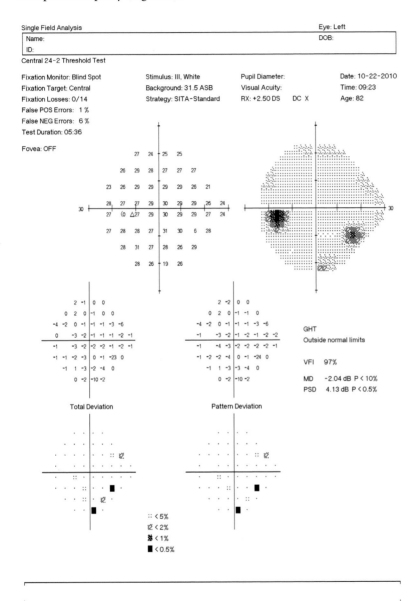

Figure 10-4
Thyroid ophthalmopathy can cause visual field defects that change rather rapidly over time. This field is from an elderly woman with radio-iodine-treated Graves' disease. The patient had diplopia, sore eyes, and rather marked exophthalmos. Visual field testing can be helpful when following patients having serious thyroid ophthalmopathy, e.g., when steroid treatment or orbital decompression is considered or being used.

Lesions of the Optic Chiasm

The optic chiasm may be damaged by pituitary adenomas, craniopharyngeomas, suprasellar meningiomas, or sometimes by aneurysms coming from the arterial circle of Willis. Crossing fibers are frequently affected first, resulting in bitemporal hemianopias. In the beginning, defects caused by infrachiasmal lesions may be limited to the superior part of the hemifield, sometimes with wedge-like defects that respect the vertical meridian. Involvement often is asymmetrical with more damage in one eye. Defects may resolve after surgery (Fig 10-5).

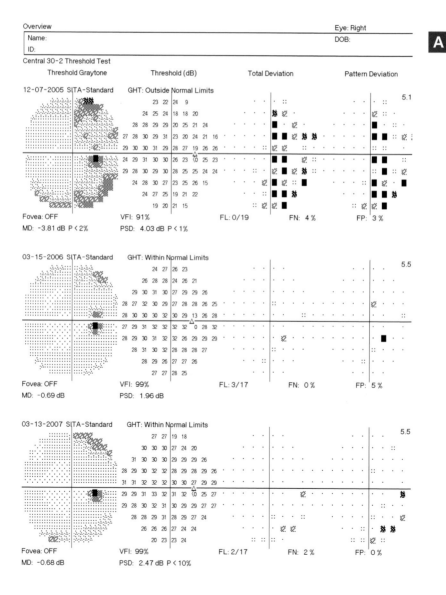

Overview

Eye: Left

Name:
ID:
DOB:

Central 30-2 Threshold Test

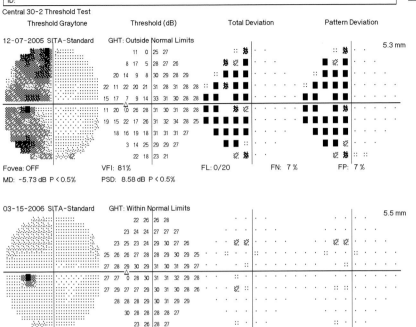

| Threshold Graytone | Threshold (dB) | Total Deviation | Pattern Deviation |

12-07-2005 SITA-Standard   GHT: Outside Normal Limits   5.3 mm

Fovea: OFF   VFI: 81%   FL: 0/20   FN: 7 %   FP: 7 %
MD: -5.73 dB P < 0.5%   PSD: 8.58 dB P < 0.5%

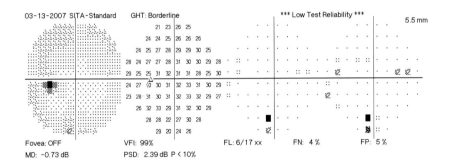

03-15-2006 SITA-Standard   GHT: Within Normal Limits   5.5 mm

Fovea: OFF   VFI: 98%   FL: 2/18   FN: 0 %   FP: 4 %
MD: -1.35 dB   PSD: 1.76 dB

03-13-2007 SITA-Standard   GHT: Borderline   *** Low Test Reliability ***   5.5 mm

Fovea: OFF   VFI: 99%   FL: 6/17 xx   FN: 4 %   FP: 5 %
MD: -0.73 dB   PSD: 2.39 dB P < 10%

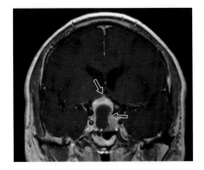

C

Figure 10-5
Bitemporal hemianopia caused by a pituitary adenoma in a 62-year-old man (A–B). The first fields show typical loss, which resolved after successful transsphenoidal surgery. The pituitary adenoma (inferior arrow) was quite large with both a sellar and a suprasellar component (C). The optic nerve chiasm can be seen stretched over the tumor (superior arrow).

Postchiasmal Lesions

Postchiasmal disease of the optic pathways results in homonymous hemianopic defects, that is, matching defects in the same visual field of both eyes. Such hemianopic defects tend to respect the vertical meridian even if they affect only part of the hemifield, for instance hemianopic wedge-like defects, quadrantanopias (Fig 10-6), and homonymous hemianopic scotomas. A large lesion involving all postchiasmal nerve fibers whether in the optic tract, the lateral geniculate body, the optic radiation, or the whole visual cortex on either the left or the right side of the brain will lead to a complete homonymous hemianopia.

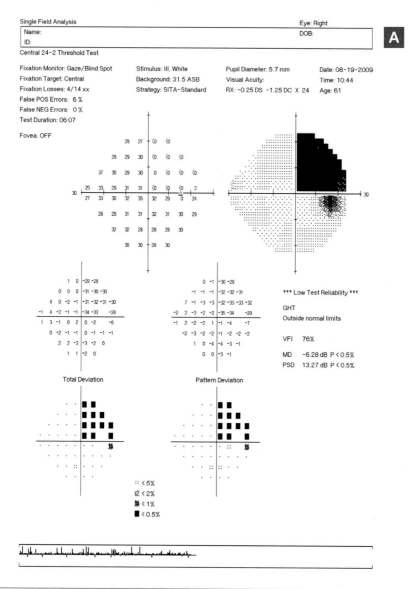

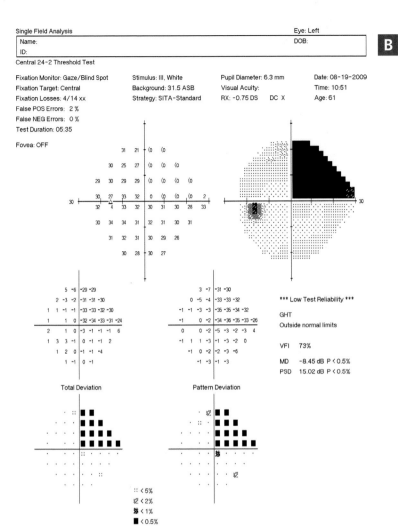

Single Field Analysis   Eye: Left

Name:	DOB:
ID:	

B

Central 24-2 Threshold Test

Fixation Monitor: Gaze/Blind Spot   Stimulus: III, White   Pupil Diameter: 6.3 mm   Date: 08-19-2009
Fixation Target: Central   Background: 31.5 ASB   Visual Acuity: Time: 10:51
Fixation Losses: 4/14 xx   Strategy: SITA-Standard   RX: -0.75 DS   DC X   Age: 61
False POS Errors: 2 %
False NEG Errors: 0 %
Test Duration: 05:35

Fovea: OFF

```
            31  21   (0  (0
         30  25  27  (0  (0  (0
      29  30  29  29  (0  (0  (0  (0
   30  27  33  32   0  (0  (0  (0   2
30 ─────────────────────────────────── 30
   32   4  33  32  30  31  30  28  33
      30  34  34  31  32  31  30  31
         31  32  31  30  29  26
            30  28  30  27
```

```
       5  -6  -29 -29                        3  -7  -31 -30
    2  -3  -2  -31 -31 -30                 0  -5  -4  -33 -33 -32
  1  1  -1  -1  -33 -33 -32 -30          -1  -1  -3  -3  -35 -35 -34 -32
  1      1   0  -32 -34 -33 -31 -24      -1       0  -2  -34 -36 -35 -33 -26
  2      1   0  -3  -1  -1  -1   6        0       0  -2  -5  -3  -2  -3   4
  1  3   3  -1   0  -1  -1   2           -1  1   1  -3  -1  -3  -2   0
     1   2   0  -1  -1  -4                -1   0  -2  -2  -1  -3  -6
        1  -1   0  -1                         -1  -3  -1  -3
```

*** Low Test Reliability ***

GHT
Outside normal limits

VFI   73%

MD   -8.45 dB P < 0.5%
PSD   15.02 dB P < 0.5%

Total Deviation   Pattern Deviation

:: < 5%
▨ < 2%
▩ < 1%
■ < 0.5%

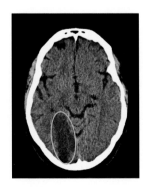

C

Figure 10-6

Homonymous quadrantanopia (A–B) caused by a cardiac embolus to the left occipital lobe in a 61-year-old woman with intermittent cardiac atrial fibrillation. The defects are absolute (there is no measurable differential light sensitivity remaining in the upper right quadrants), and the defects respect the vertical and horizontal meridians perfectly. As expected, the VFI indices are both close to 75%. The infarct is visible on MRI (the darker area within the blue oval) (C).

Congruity—the degree to which defects in the two eyes match or slightly differ—may be used to help localize the lesion. Postchiasmal visual field defects usually are more congruous when they are caused by lesions situated further back toward the occipital cortex. Damage to the visual cortex itself should in principle result in perfectly matching defects in the two eyes.

11

Visual Field Loss
in Retinal Diseases

PERIMETRY IS NOT THE most important tool for diagnosing or monitoring retinal disease, because most lesions are visible on fundus examination or imaging. However, retinal disease sometimes is identified because of field defects found accidentally, e.g. in the routine management of glaucoma patients. Perhaps more importantly, multiple diseases can coexist in the same eye, such as glaucoma and retinal vascular disease, making it necessary to identify which disease is causing the observed field loss. In any case, a working knowledge of how retinal disease can affect the visual field is necessary in clinical care.

A common field defect caused by retinal disease is the central scotoma associated with age-related macular degeneration. In many cases, just a few central test point locations may be affected on a 24-2 or 30-2 test (Fig 11-1), but higher density 10-2 testing will show a more detailed picture. Patients having deep central scotomas who need perimetric examination, e.g., because of concurrent glaucoma can be tested quite effectively using the Humphrey perimeter's large diamond fixation target instead of the standard fixation light emitting diode (LED), even if visual acuity is very low.[76]

Central serous retinopathy also results in reduced central visual function, and therefore in central scotomas. Visual acuity is often only moderately reduced, and the resulting field loss may be discrete and apparent only in probability maps.

Retinochoroiditis may cause arcuate or wedge-like defects that can be mistaken for glaucomatous lesions (Fig 11-2). The cause of the problem is identified, of course, when lesions are seen during ophthalmoscopy. The visual field findings themselves may offer some clues that can help refine the diagnosis. Field defects caused by retinal lesions frequently are deep and sharply defined, and they tend to show much less variability from test to test than comparable glaucomatous lesions.

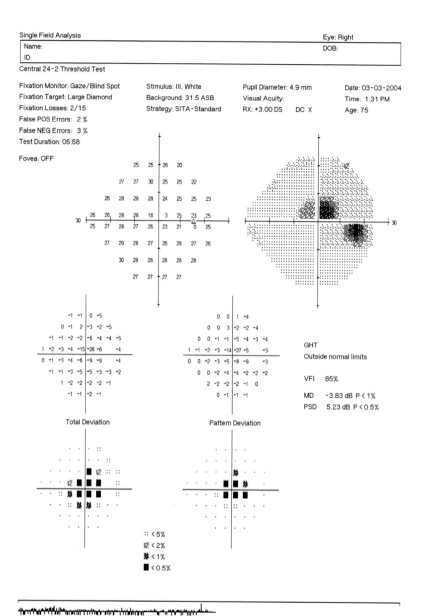

Figure 11-1

Visual field loss caused by advanced age-related macular degeneration (ARMD). The patient was tested because an optic disc hemorrhage had been documented in this eye raising a suspicion of glaucoma. Visual acuity was only finger counting at one-half meter, and there was considerable atrophy in and around the macula. The field test result helped exclude potentially important glaucoma damage in this eye. This case also demonstrates that successful perimetry is possible in ARMD eyes, even if visual acuity is poor. Patients with deep central scotomas should be instructed to center their gaze in the center between the four LEDs that make up the large diamond fixation target of the perimeter.

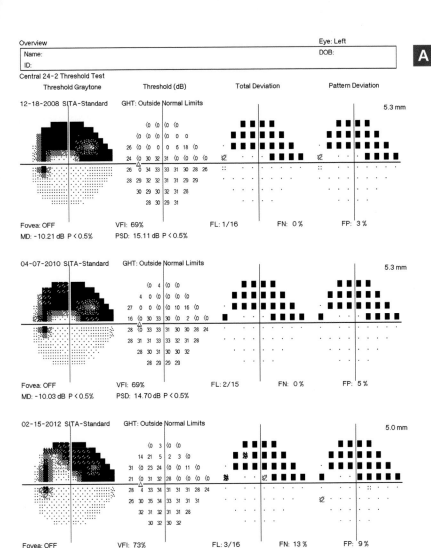

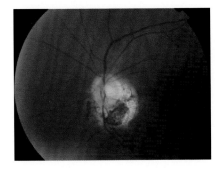

Figure 11-2

Retinochoroiditis destroys retinal nerve fiber bundles and can therefore result in arcuate field defects of the same type as those in glaucoma (A). Defects are deep and can be remarkably reproducible, often with sharp borders. The diagnosis is unlikely to be missed, especially if the lesion is located close to the disc, as in this case (B); sometimes, less obvious cases may be classified as glaucomatous, in the absence of careful fundus examination.

Field loss from diabetic retinopathy often is relative and multifocal, giving the field a mottled appearance. Subtle losses have been reported in mild background retinopathy,[57, 130] while clear perimetric defects are more common in moderate and advanced stages (43 and higher in the Early Treatment of Diabetic Retinopathy Study [ETDRS] scale) (Fig 11-3).[131] Central (10-2) SWAP testing has been reported to be

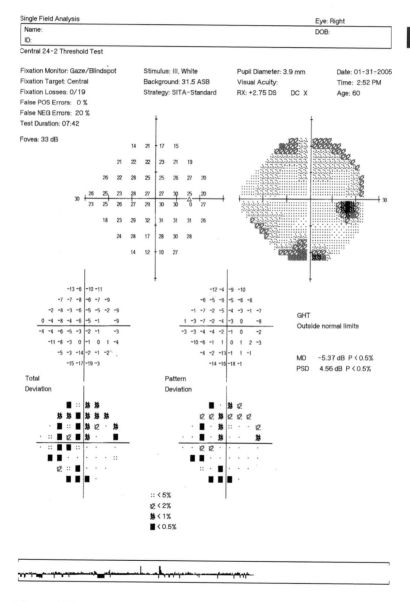

Figure 11-3
Diabetic retinopathy can cause field defects, often of a patchy nature (A).

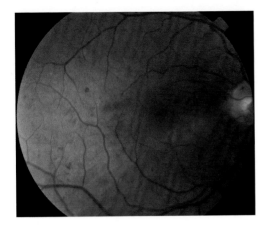

B

Figure 11-3 **continued**
**The field is from an eye with
moderate nonproliferative
retinopathy (B).**

more sensitive than standard white-on-white perimetry to damage in the foveal and perifoveal capillary network.[55, 57]

Retinal detachments and retinoschises cause field defects, but since such defects commonly are located in the peripheral field, they are often not seen in conventional central visual field testing. Retinal detachments will typically cause relative defects, while retinoschises naturally produce absolute defects with sharp borders, because the inner and outer retinal segments are split apart.

Sometimes visual field examination becomes important in the evaluation of a patient with retinal disease, or conversely, the results of the visual field examination may raise the possibility of a retinal diagnosis. Typical field loss in retinal disease is circular and initially located in the midperiphery, but can progress to tunnel vision. Therefore, searching for visual field loss caused by retinitis pigmentosa is one of the few clinical situations where a standard 24-2 or 30-2 threshold test may not be the best choice. A suprathreshold test that includes peripheral field may be preferable, particularly because field defects there often are deep and easily identified.

Of course, retinal vascular occlusions are primarily diagnosed with ophthalmoscopy, but it is important, such as when following patients with glaucoma, to understand what sort of defects can be caused by retinal vascular disease. Arterial occlusions typically result in absolute field defects, while venous occlusions produce highly variable field loss. Thus, eyes with small branch vein occlusions may have entirely normal fields, while central vein occlusions may sometimes be associated with profound and widespread field loss.

12

Artifactual Test Results

PERIMETRIC TEST RESULTS CAN sometimes falsely suggest that a normal eye has an artifactually abnormal field. Fortunately, the patterns of such artifactual field loss are often characteristic and easily recognized. False patterns may be caused by ptosis, prominent brows, misaligned correction lenses, lack of proper patient instruction and supervision, patient inattention, or patient anxiety.

Many false patterns occur in the more peripheral part of the tested field. Therefore, artifactual test results are less common in 24-2 fields compared to 30-2 tests. It is also fortunate that many of these effects can be remedied by more careful patient instruction and supervision.

The Untrained Patient and Perimetric Learning

Perhaps 10% of patients show slightly decreased visual field sensitivity on their first perimetry test.[103–105, 132] However, in our experience, these learning effects seldom are large enough to require that the field be discarded and re-done, except perhaps in clinical trials. Such initial fields typically show reduced sensitivity in the midperiphery, 20° to 30° from fixation, while the very central part of the field appears to be normal. Midperipheral constriction due to inexperience usually is less apparent in the smaller 24-2 test point pattern than in the larger 30-2 pattern (Fig 12-1). If the test is repeated, the results usually will improve, especially if the patient has been carefully reinstructed and supervised. However, a minority of patients may require more than one testing session before producing reliable results.

Experience gained with one type of perimetric testing may not be transferable to another test modality, e.g., in switching from Frequency Doubling Technology (FDT) testing to standard Humphrey perimetry.

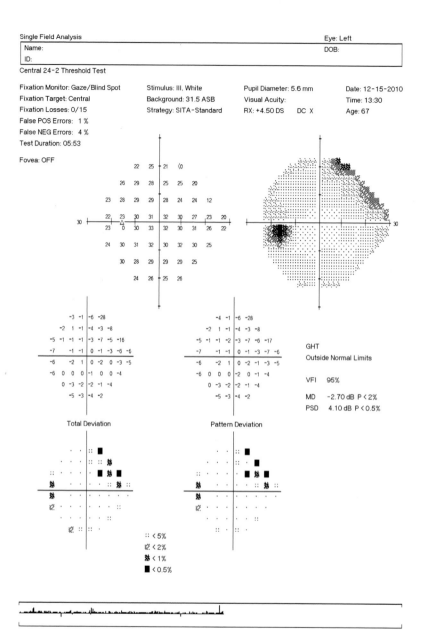

Figure 12-1

A minority of patients may not produce entirely representative field test results on their first test (A). In such cases it is typically the most peripheral test point locations that are somewhat depressed. Nowadays, when SITA 24-2 testing is more common, learning effects usually are small and of little clinical importance, as in this early glaucoma case in which the second test (B) shows only modest improvement.

Single Field Analysis	Eye: Left
Name:	DOB:
ID:	

B

Central 24-2 Threshold Test

Fixation Monitor: Gaze/Blind Spot
Fixation Target: Central
Fixation Losses: 4/16 xx
False POS Errors: 5 %
False NEG Errors: 4 %
Test Duration: 05:53

Fovea: OFF

Stimulus: III, White
Background: 31.5 ASB
Strategy: SITA-Standard

Pupil Diameter: 5.6 mm
Visual Acuity:
RX: +4.50 DS   DC X

Date: 04-14-2011
Time: 14.18
Age: 67

```
              19  22  20  19
          24  25  24  27  27  19
      28  25  25  30  30  27  26  15
      24  19  30  32  32  29  25  23  24
30 ---------△------------------------------- 30
      26  2   29  33  32  31  30  30  24
      23  30  33  31  32  31  31  30
          27  30  28  28  30  28
              24  26  24  24
```

Total Deviation

```
      -6  -4 | -6  -7
   -3  -3  -5 | -2  -2  -9
 0  -4  -5   0 | -1  -3  -4 -13
-5  -1   0   0 | -2  -5  -6  -2
   -3      -2   1 | 0  -1  -1   1   2
-6   0   3   0 | 0   0   1   2
   -3   0  -2 | -2   0  -1
      -5  -3 | -5  -4
```

Pattern Deviation

```
      -6  -4 | -7  -7
   -3  -3  -5 | -2  -2  -9
 0  -4  -5  -1 | -1  -4  -4 -13
-5  -1   0   0 | -3  -5  -6  -2
   -3      -2   1 | -1  -1  -1   1  -2
-7  -1   2   0 | 0   0   0   1
   -3  -1  -2 | -3  -1  -2
      -5  -4 | -6  -4
```

*** Low Test Reliability ***

GHT
Outside Normal Limits

VFI   96%

MD   -2.15 dB P < 5%
PSD   2.89 dB P < 2%

:: < 5%
▨ < 2%
▨ < 1%
■ < 0.5%

Lid Artifacts

Partial ptosis is quite common and frequently produces artifactual field defects, and such defects often appear to be most obvious on the grayscale printout. That this type of pattern is normal and not uncommon may be obvious from the probability maps, where slight ptosis often does not result in readings indicating high statistical significance (Fig 12-2). While usually not necessary, the upper lid may be temporarily

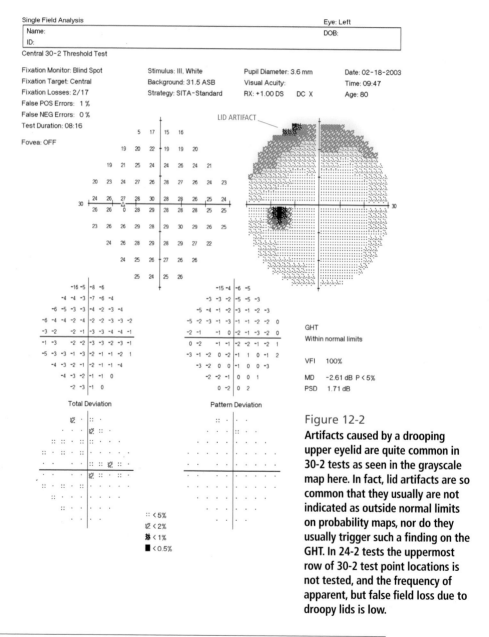

Figure 12-2

Artifacts caused by a drooping upper eyelid are quite common in 30-2 tests as seen in the grayscale map here. In fact, lid artifacts are so common that they usually are not indicated as outside normal limits on probability maps, nor do they usually trigger such a finding on the GHT. In 24-2 tests the uppermost row of 30-2 test point locations is not tested, and the frequency of apparent, but false field loss due to droopy lids is low.

elevated, for instance with surgical tape, in order to rule out other possible causes of such superior field defects. Also ptosis artifacts are, of course, less commonly seen in 24-2 tests than in 30-2 tests.

Trial Lens Artifacts

In strongly hyperopic patients, trial lenses may magnify the visual field to the point that peripheral parts of the 30-2 test pattern are obscured by the lens rim or the lens holder (Fig 12-3). More moderate positive lens corrections will simply increase the likelihood that small misalignments of the eye relative to the lens holder will result in blockage of peripheral test points. Even weak lenses may create artifactual field loss if the patient is significantly misaligned or has moved back from the lens. Trial lens artifacts are less common in 24-2 tests than in 30-2 tests.

These patterns usually are easy to recognize if appearing in otherwise normal fields, as they most often involve a ring of peripheral points having low sensitivities, producing an organized false defect with sharp borders. However, lens artifacts can be difficult to differentiate from real progression in eyes with more significant loss. Six mm of decentration of the eye relative to the lens center may produce a trial lens artifact when using a +3 D correction at a vertex distance of 15 mm. With a +10 D lens, less than 3 mm of decentration can be allowed if the vertex distance is 15 mm. More decentration can be tolerated at shorter vertex distances and less at larger vertex distances. Thus, it is generally good practice to place trial lenses as close to the eye as is practical, with the limiting factor often being the brow or the eyelashes. Naturally, artifactual patterns caused by correction lens are likely to disappear upon further testing if the patient is carefully reinstructed and well supervised.

Name:

ID:

DOB:

Central 30-2 Threshold Test

Fixation Monitor: Gaze/Blind Spot	Stimulus: III, White	Pupil Diameter:	Date: 07-04-2012
Fixation Target: Central	Background: 31.5 ASB	Visual Acuity:	Time: 13:44
Fixation Losses: 0/16	Strategy: SITA-Fast	RX: +8.00 DS DC X	Age: 59
False POS Errors: 0 %			
False NEG Errors: 9 %			
Test Duration: 08:20			
Fovea: OFF			

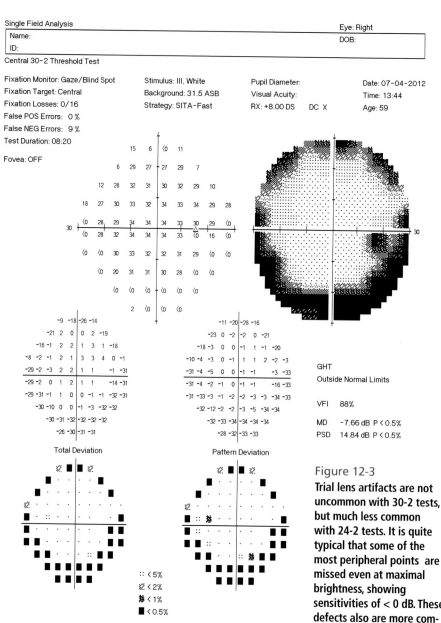

GHT

Outside Normal Limits

VFI   88%

MD   -7.66 dB P < 0.5%

PSD   14.84 dB P < 0.5%

Total Deviation

Pattern Deviation

:: < 5%

⊠ < 2%

▓ < 1%

■ < 0.5%

Figure 12-3

Trial lens artifacts are not uncommon with 30-2 tests, but much less common with 24-2 tests. It is quite typical that some of the most peripheral points are missed even at maximal brightness, showing sensitivities of < 0 dB. These defects also are more common in hyperopic eyes when strong plus trial lenses are used for testing (+7.58 D in this case), but they can occur also in emmetropic patients if the tested eye is decentered, or if the trial lens is situated too far forward from the eye.

The Inattentive Patient and the Cloverleaf Field

The cloverleaf field is a very characteristic artifactual pattern associated with patient inattention (Fig 12-4). This pattern occurs when the patient has responded more or less normally during the first part of the test, but then given up, often as a result of misunderstanding or poor supervision. The patient may have asked the operator for a rest, or whether the test was over, or how to respond. If the operator was no longer in the room the patient may not have known what to do—and may have chosen to do nothing.

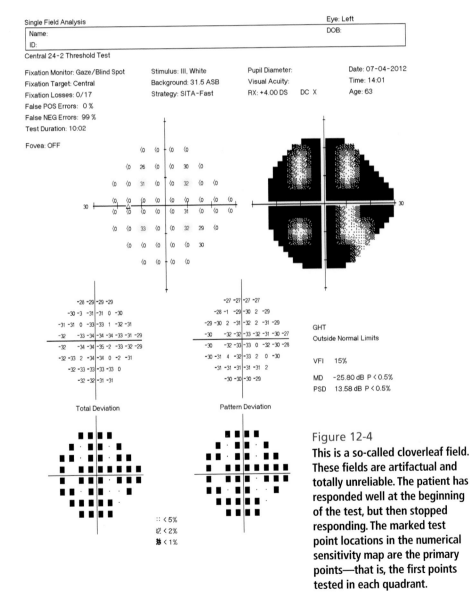

Figure 12-4

This is a so-called cloverleaf field. These fields are artifactual and totally unreliable. The patient has responded well at the beginning of the test, but then stopped responding. The marked test point locations in the numerical sensitivity map are the primary points—that is, the first points tested in each quadrant.

If you see many cloverleaf fields in your practice, your staff may need more training in how to instruct and supervise perimetric patients.

The Trigger-Happy Field

Some patients, particularly if they are anxious, may press the response button even when the stimulus is too dim to be seen, resulting in large numbers of false responses. False positive responses can affect the test result in a number of ways. Often, "trigger-happy" responses will artificially push up measured threshold values at some test points to levels that no human can see, resulting in patches of abnormally light or even entirely white areas on the grayscale presentation (Fig 12-5). In such cases, the false-positive catch trial rate is likely to be elevated and the Pattern Deviation probability plot may artifactually show more defective points than are seen in the Total Deviation plot. The Glaucoma Hemifield Test may also display the Abnormally High Sensitivity message. As usual, the remedy is to carefully reinstruct the patient and to retest. A less obvious example of a trigger-happy field is shown in Fig 5-4.

Sudden and Unexpected Change

Diseases followed over time with repeated visual fields will often show slowly progressive change. The most common example is glaucoma, of course, but there are many other such conditions, for instance, pituitary tumors and retinal dystrophies. Large observed differences between two consecutive fields often are not the result of progression of the original disease but instead are associated with some new condition. For example, a sudden and large change in a glaucoma patient may be due to a stroke (Fig 12-6), or perhaps retinal vascular occlusion. Stroke can be suspected when the new field loss respects the vertical meridian, at least to some extent. However, this may be difficult to detect if there already is considerable glaucomatous field loss. If the damage is postchiasmal there will be evidence of sudden and similar worsening in both of the patient's visual fields. In contrast, sudden progression caused by retinal vascular catastrophes will be unilateral.

In any case, it is wise to consider and rule out other unexpected disease any time that large and sudden apparent field progression is found when following patients who have chronic disease.

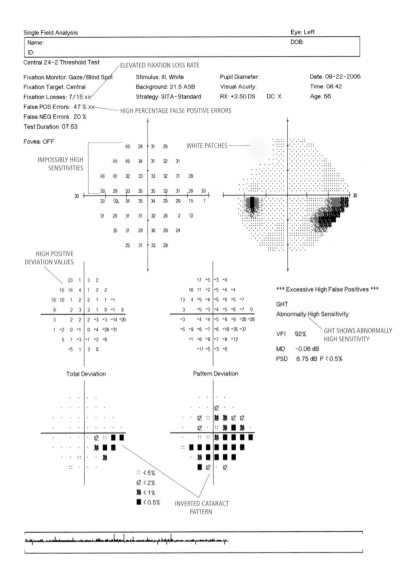

Figure 12-5

This so-called "trigger-happy" field is the result of a test with a high percentage of false positive responses, in which the patient frequently pressed the response button without perceiving a stimulus. There are at least five distinct indicators of a high level of false positive responses in this report: 1) The percentage of False Positive Errors is high and has resulted in a message saying "Excessive High False Positives." 2) Blind spot check errors are elevated. 3) Measured threshold sensitivities are above normal physiological limits at many test point locations, with high positive values in the numerical Total Deviation map, and white patches in the grayscale map. 4) The GHT message shows "Abnormally High Sensitivity." 5) There is an "inverted cataract pattern" in the probability maps, in which there are many more significant points in the Pattern Deviation probability map than in the total deviation probability map. A sixth sign is absent in this example, but sometimes is seen, in which the blind spot is not indicated on the grayscale plot.

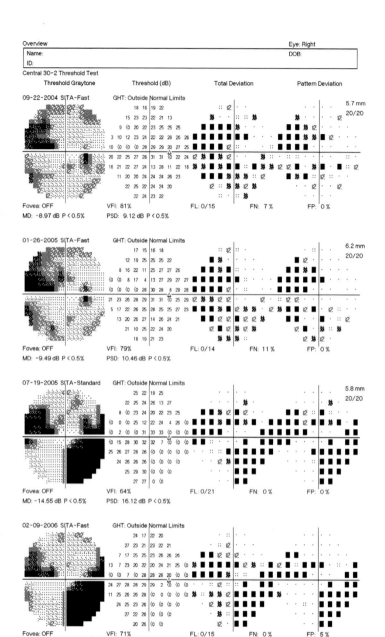

Figure 12-6

This is a field series from both eyes of a patient with bilateral glaucoma damage who suffered a stroke (A–B). Sudden large changes in the field test results of glaucoma patients frequently have nonglaucomatous causes. In this case the diagnosis was uncomplicated, because both fields developed additional congruent hemianopic damage.

Name: Eye: Left
                                                          DOB:
ID:

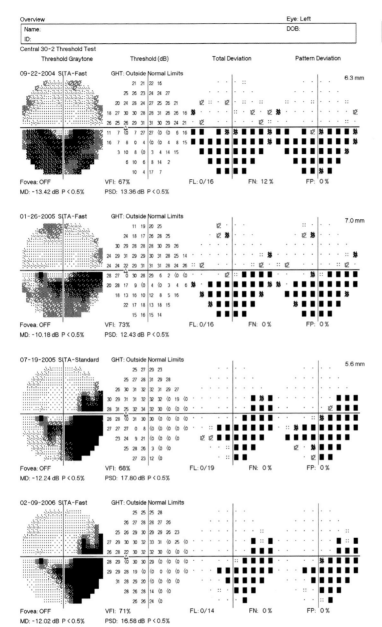

Central 30-2 Threshold Test

| Threshold Graytone | Threshold (dB) | Total Deviation | Pattern Deviation |

09-22-2004 SITA-Fast — GHT: Outside Normal Limits — 6.3 mm
Fovea: OFF
VFI: 67%   FL: 0/16   FN: 12 %   FP: 0 %
MD: -13.42 dB P < 0.5%   PSD: 13.36 dB P < 0.5%

01-26-2005 SITA-Fast — GHT: Outside Normal Limits — 7.0 mm
Fovea: OFF
VFI: 73%   FL: 0/16   FN: 0 %   FP: 0 %
MD: -10.18 dB P < 0.5%   PSD: 12.43 dB P < 0.5%

07-19-2005 SITA-Standard — GHT: Outside Normal Limits — 5.6 mm
Fovea: OFF
VFI: 68%   FL: 0/19   FN: 0 %   FP: 0 %
MD: -12.24 dB P < 0.5%   PSD: 17.80 dB P < 0.5%

02-09-2006 SITA-Fast — GHT: Outside Normal Limits — 5.6 mm
Fovea: OFF
VFI: 71%   FL: 0/14   FN: 0 %   FP: 0 %
MD: -12.02 dB P < 0.5%   PSD: 16.58 dB P < 0.5%

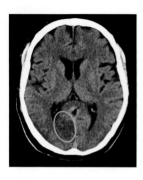

C

Figure 12-6 **continued**
The infarct of the left occipital lobe is clearly visible in the CT scan (the slightly darker area within the blue oval) (C).

13

Perimeter Design

THE HUMPHREY PERIMETER CONSISTS of four basic elements: the bowl or projection surface, the optical system, the computer system, and the patient interface. In designing the HFA, our overall goal was to combine accurate and consistent perimetric testing with ergonomic features that provide as much patient comfort as possible.

The Bowl

The bowl of the HFA II is a patented, aspherical, or bullet-shaped white surface upon which stimuli are projected (Fig 13-1). This is a departure from earlier hemispherical designs, such as the original Goldmann perimeter, and was adopted because it improves patient ergonomics and reduces instrument size. All Humphrey perimeters built since 1995 have this kind of bowl.

The distance from the eye to the center of the bowl is 30 centimeters—the same as the original Goldmann perimeter. The amount of asphericity was chosen so that the surface departs insignificantly from the traditional spherical shape in the central 30°, thus providing very close agreement between modern HFA test results and those of the original Humphrey perimeter, now known as HFA I.[133] This curvature also was chosen to ensure that the refractive correction needed for clear vision in the center of the bowl is proper even at the edge of the central visual field. Stimulus brightness outside the central 30° is adjusted to compensate for the difference in testing distance between the aspherical bowl and

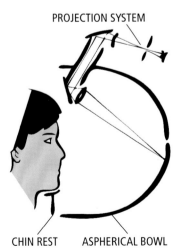

PROJECTION SYSTEM

CHIN REST   ASPHERICAL BOWL

Figure 13-1
The bowl of the HFA is aspherical and bullet-shaped, which makes the perimeter more compact and ergonomical without compromising the physical requirements of perimetric testing.

traditional hemispheres. While this adjustment is only an approximation, the amount of compensation is not large compared to typical measurement precision.

The bowl surface is textured to provide an almost perfectly matte finish; this is known as a Lambertian surface. Lambertian surfaces are the opposite of mirrors. They provide almost no direct or specular reflections but instead scatter light diffusely and equally in all directions. Thus, stimuli projected on this surface will seem equally bright regardless of viewing angle.

The Optical System

The HFA II optical system projects stimuli of known size and brightness in a known location for a known amount of time. Stimuli are projected onto a bowl having a standard brightness. All five standard Goldmann stimulus Sizes (I through V) are available, although most testing is done with the Size III. Stimuli are presented by aiming an optical projector at the particular location to be tested, adjusting a set of neutral density filters to obtain the correct stimulus brightness, and then opening a shutter for a standard time, usually 200 milliseconds. Mechanical motions are constantly monitored by built-in electronics, in order to help ensure that calibration accuracy is maintained throughout testing.

Background brightness—the brightness of the bowl surface itself—is checked at the beginning of each test, and constantly during testing in order to adjust for any changes in room illumination. Stimulus bulb brightness is checked every time the instrument is started up. Stimulus brightness is then finely adjusted just before each stimulus is presented, based upon the local background brightness measured at each test location. This fine adjustment is done with the goal of correcting stimulus contrast for any local variations in bowl brightness, such as might be caused by shadows falling on the bowl from an open door.

The Computer and Connectivity

The HFA's computer controls instrument calibration, error checking, testing strategy, STATPAC data analysis, printing, and electronic transmission and storage of test results. In some cases, data storage and printing may be done using a separate computer. The graphical user interface may be controlled via the instrument's touch screen, or via mouse and keyboard.

As with all computers, HFA is vulnerable to data loss, and all clinical data must be safeguarded by frequent backup. Current HFA models may be networked via Ethernet connection, using ZEISS's FORUM software (Fig 13-2). FORUM facilitates transmittal of results to a centralized database that can be shared with other

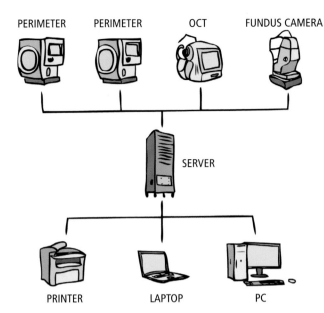

PERIMETER   PERIMETER   OCT   FUNDUS CAMERA

SERVER

PRINTER   LAPTOP   PC

Figure 13-2
ZEISS FORUM software facilitates connection of multiple HFAs and other DICOM-compatible products to a common server, allowing storage and backup of test results and reports, and presentation of structural and functional test results in a single report.

Humphrey perimeters and also can store results from other ZEISS products and other DICOM-compatible (Digital Imaging and Communications in Medicine) devices. Backup of the centralized database may then be managed in the context of the practice's general data backup processes.

FORUM allows remote electronic presentation of test reports, for example on monitors located in each consulting room. FORUM also allows production of reports in which Cirrus HD-OCT and HFA test results are combined into a single integrated presentation.

Patient Ergonomics

Patient comfort is significantly more important for perimeters than for instruments such as autorefractors or even slit lamps. Autorefraction may take only a few seconds and does not require the patient to concentrate on properly performing a task. Slit lamp examination may take longer than autorefraction, but usually is brief compared to threshold visual field testing of both eyes.

Proper ergonomic design improves patient satisfaction, alertness, and compliance, and for all these reasons, HFA was designed to maximize patient comfort. The bullet bowl minimizes instrument size, and allows patients to be rolled right up to the perimeter and to be tested while sitting comfortably upright. Instruments having larger bowls are bulkier, and some patients may not be able to reach the chinrest without having to lean forward uncomfortably. The HFA instrument table was designed to allow wheelchair patients to be rolled into testing position, again without having to lean uncomfortably forward or to stretch to reach the chinrest.

The patient response button was designed for maximum comfort for elderly patients. In those whose fingers have been weakened by, for example arthritis, the button can even be pressed with a closed hand.

References

1. Kutzko KE, Brito CF, Wall M. Effect of instructions on conventional automated perimetry. *Invest Ophthalmol Vis Sci.* 2000; 41(7): 2006–13.

2. Keltner JL, Johnson CA, Cello KE, Bandermann SE, Fan J, Levine RA, et al. Visual field quality control in the Ocular Hypertension Treatment Study (OHTS). *J Glaucoma.* 2007; 16(8): 665–9.

3. Heuer DK, Anderson DR, Feuer WJ, Gressel MG. The influence of refraction accuracy on automated perimetric threshold measurements. *Ophthalmology.* 1987; 94(12): 1550–3.

4. Barkana Y, Gerber Y, Mora R, Liebmann JM, Ritch R. Effect of eye testing order on automated perimetry results using the Swedish Interactive Threshold Algorithm standard 24-2. *Arch Ophthalmol.* 2006; 124(6): 781–4.

5. Van Coevorden RE, Mills RP, Chen YY, Barnebey HS. Continuous visual field test supervision may not always be necessary. *Ophthalmology.* 1999; 106(1): 178–81.

6. Kramer BC, Musch DC, Niziol LM, Weizer JS. Reliability of simultaneous visual field testing. *Ophthalmology.* 2012; 119(2): 304–7.

7. Ramachandran VS, Gregory RL. Perceptual filling in of artificially induced scotomas in human vision. *Nature.* 1991; 350(6320): 699–702.

8. Das A, Gilbert CD. Long-range horizontal connections and their role in cortical reorganization revealed by optical recording of cat primary visual cortex. *Nature.* 1995; 375(6534): 780–4.

9. Safran AB, Landis T. From cortical plasticity to unawareness of visual field defects. *J Neuroophthalmol.* 1999; 19(2): 84–8.

10. Hoste AM. New insights into the subjective perception of visual field defects. *Bull Soc Belge Ophtalmol.* 2003; (287): 65–71.

11. Lynn JR. Examination of the visual field in glaucoma. *Invest Ophthalmol.* 1969; 8(1): 76–84.

12. Heijl A. Automatic perimetry in glaucoma visual field screening. A clinical study. Albrecht Von Graefes Arch Klin Exp Ophthalmol. 1976; 200(1): 21–37.

13. Gramer E, Pröll M, Krieglstein GK. [Reproducibility of central visual field testing using kinetic or computerized static perimetry (author's transl)]. *Klin Monbl Augenheilkd.* 1980; 176(3): 374–84.

14. Gloor B, Sturmer J, Vokt B. [What new knowledge has automated perimetry with the Octopus brought on glaucomatous visual field changes?]. *Klin Monbl Augenheilkd.* 1984; 184(4): 249–53.

15. Herbolzheimer WG. [Computer program controlled perimetry, its advantages and disadvantages]. *Klin Monbl Augenheilkd.* 1986; 189(4): 270–7.

16. Katz J, Tielsch JM, Quigley HA, Sommer A. Automated perimetry detects visual field loss before manual Goldmann perimetry. *Ophthalmology.* 1995; 102(1): 21–6.

17. Sloan LL. The Tubinger perimeter of Harms and Aulhorn. Recommended procedures and supplementary equipment. *Arch Ophthalmol.* 1971; 86(6): 612–22.

18. Sample PA, Dannheim F, Artes PH, Dietzsch J, Henson D, Johnson CA, et al. Imaging and Perimetry Society standards and guidelines. *Optom Vis Sci.* 2011; 88(1): 4–7.

19. Kunimatsu S, Suzuki Y, Shirato S, Araie M. Usefulness of gaze tracking during perimetry in glaucomatous eyes. *Jpn J Ophthalmol.* 2000; 44(2): 190–1.

20. Heijl A, Krakau CE. An automatic static perimeter, design and pilot study. *Acta Ophthalmol* (Copen h). 1975; 53(3): 293–310.

21. Mills RP, Barnebey HS, Migliazzo CV, Li Y. Does saving time using FASTPAC or suprathreshold testing reduce quality of visual fields? *Ophthalmology.* 1994; 101(9): 1596–603.

22. Alexander LJ, Corliss DA, Vinson C, Williams J, Casser L, Fingeret M, et al. Clinical implications of intra- and inter-reader agreement in four different automated visual fields. *J Am Optom Assoc.* 1995; 66(11): 681–92.

23. Khoury JM, Donahue SP, Lavin PJ, Tsai JC. Comparison of 24-2 and 30-2 perimetry in glaucomatous and nonglaucomatous optic neuropathies. *J Neuroophthalmol.* 1999; 19(2): 100–8.

24. Heijl A, Bengtsson B, Chauhan BC, Lieberman MF, Cunliffe I, Hyman L, et al. A comparison of visual field progression criteria of 3 major glaucoma trials in early manifest glaucoma trial patients. *Ophthalmology.* 2008; 115(9): 1557–65.

25. Caprioli J, Spaeth GL. Static threshold examination of the peripheral nasal visual field in glaucoma. *Arch Ophthalmol.* 1985; 103(8): 1150–4.

26. Stewart WC, Shields MB. The peripheral visual field in glaucoma: reevaluation in the age of automated perimetry. *Surv Ophthalmol.* 1991; 36(1): 59–69.

27. Hard-Boberg AL, Wirtschafeter JD. Evaluating the usefulness in neuro-ophthalmology of visual field examination peripheral to 30 degrees. In: Heijl A, Greve EL, editors. *Sixth International Visual Field Symposium, Santa Margherita Ligure, 1984.* Dordrecht: Dr W Junk Publishers; 1985; 197–206.

28. Keltner JL, Johnson CA, Spurr JO, Beck RW. Comparison of central and peripheral visual field properties in the optic neuritis treatment trial. *Am J Ophthalmol.* 1999; 128(5): 543–53.

29. Bengtsson B, Olsson J, Heijl A, Rootzen H. A new generation of algorithms for computerized threshold perimetry, SITA. *Acta Ophthalmol* Scand. 1997; 75(4): 368–75.

30. Bengtsson B, Heijl A. SITA Fast, a new rapid perimetric threshold test. Description of methods and evaluation in patients with manifest and suspect glaucoma. *Acta Ophthalmol* Scand. 1998; 76(4): 431–7.

31. Bengtsson B, Heijl A. Normal intersubject threshold variability and normal limits of the SITA SWAP and full threshold SWAP perimetric programs. *Invest Ophthalmol Vis Sci.* 2003; 44(11): 5029–34.

32. Bengtsson B, Heijl A, Olsson J. Evaluation of a new threshold visual field strategy, SITA, in normal subjects. Swedish Interactive Thresholding Algorithm. *Acta Ophthalmol* Scand. 1998; 76(2): 165–9.

33. Bengtsson B, Heijl A. Evaluation of a new perimetric threshold strategy, SITA, in patients with manifest and suspect glaucoma. *Acta Ophthalmol Scand.* 1998; 76(3): 268–72.

34. Tsuji A, Inazumi K, Yamamoto T, Kitazawa Y. [Evaluation of the Swedish Interactive Thresholding Algorithm, a new thresholding algorithm, of the Humphrey field analyzer in normal subjects]. *Nihon Ganka Gakkai Zasshi.* 1998; 102(6): 359–64.

35. Bengtsson B HA. Sensitivity to glaucomatous visual field loss in full threshold, SITA Standard and SITA Fast tests. In: Heijl A, editor. *Perimetry Update 1998/99.* Amsterdam, Milano, Berkeley: Kugler Ghedini; 1999: 3–7.

36. Bengtsson B, Heijl A. Comparing significance and magnitude of glaucomatous visual field defects using the SITA and Full Threshold strategies. *Acta Ophthalmol* Scand. 1999; 77(2): 143–6.

37. Bengtsson B, Heijl A. Inter-subject variability and normal limits of the SITA Standard, SITA Fast, and the Humphrey Full Threshold computerized perimetry strategies, SITA STATPAC. *Acta Ophthalmol* Scand. 1999; 77(2): 125–9.

38. Shirato S, Inoue R, Fukushima K, Suzuki Y. Clinical evaluation of SITA: a new family of perimetric testing strategies. *Graefes Arch Clin Exp Ophthalmol.* 1999; 237(1): 29–34.

39. Sekhar GC, Naduvilath TJ, Lakkai M, Jayakumar AJ, Pandi GT, Mandal AK, et al. Sensitivity of Swedish interactive threshold algorithm compared with standard full threshold algorithm in Humphrey visual field testing. *Ophthalmology.* 2000; 107(7): 1303–8.

40. Artes PH, Iwase A, Ohno Y, Kitazawa Y, Chauhan BC. Properties of perimetric threshold estimates from Full Threshold, SITA Standard, and SITA Fast strategies. *Invest Ophthalmol Vis Sci.* 2002; 43(8): 2654–9.

41. Budenz DL, Rhee P, Feuer WJ, McSoley J, Johnson CA, Anderson DR. Comparison of glaucomatous visual field defects using standard full threshold and Swedish interactive threshold algorithms. *Arch Ophthalmol.* 2002; 120(9): 1136–41.

42. Budenz DL, Rhee P, Feuer WJ, McSoley J, Johnson CA, Anderson DR. Sensitivity and specificity of the Swedish interactive threshold algorithm for glaucomatous visual field defects. *Ophthalmology.* 2002; 109(6): 1052–8.

43. Marmor MF, Kellner U, Lai TY, Lyons JS, Mieler WF. Revised recommendations on screening for chloroquine and hydroxychloroquine retinopathy. *Ophthalmology.* 2011; 118(2): 415–22.

44. Disability Evaluation Under Social Security (Blue Book August 2010) In: Administration UGSS, editor. http://www.ssa.gov/disability/ professionals/bluebook/; 2010.

45. McKnight AJ, Shinar D, Hilburn B. The visual and driving performance of monocular and binocular heavy-duty truck drivers. *Accid Anal Prev.* 1991; 23(4): 225–37.

46. Crabb DP, Smith ND, Rauscher FG, Chisholm CM, Barbur JL, Edgar DF, et al. Exploring eye movements in patients with glaucoma when viewing a driving scene. *PLoS One.* 2010; 5(3): e9710.

47. Anderson DR, Patella V.M. *Automated Static Perimetry.* 3rd ed. St Louis: Mosby; 1999; 820–9.

48. Cahill KV, Bradley EA, Meyer DR, Custer PL, Holck DE, Marcet MM, et al. *Functional indications for upper eyelid ptosis and blepharoplasty surgery:* a report by the American Academy of Ophthalmology. Ophthalmology. 2011; 118(12): 2510–7.

49. Cahill KV, Burns JA, Weber PA. The effect of blepharoptosis on the field of vision. *Ophthal Plast Reconstr Surg.* 1987; 3(3): 121–5.

50. Hacker HD, Hollsten DA. Investigation of automated perimetry in the evaluation of patients for upper lid blepharoplasty. *Ophthal Plast Reconstr Surg.* 1992; 8(4): 250–5.

51. Lewis RA, Johnson CA, Adams AJ. Automated perimetry and short wavelength sensitivity in patients with asymmetric intraocular pressures. *Graefes Arch Clin Exp Ophthalmol.* 1993; 231(5): 274–8.

52. Sample PA, Taylor JD, Martinez GA, Lusky M, Weinreb RN. Short-wavelength color visual fields in glaucoma suspects at risk. *Am J Ophthalmol.* 1993; 115(2): 225–33.

53. Bengtsson B, Heijl A. Diagnostic sensitivity of fast blue-yellow and standard automated perimetry in early glaucoma: a comparison between different test programs. *Ophthalmology.* 2006; 113(7): 1092–7.

54. van der Schoot J, Reus NJ, Colen TP, Lemij HG. The ability of short-wavelength automated perimetry to predict conversion to glaucoma. *Ophthalmology.* 2010; 117(1): 30–4.

55. Remky A, Arend O, Hendricks S. Short-wavelength automated perimetry and capillary density in early diabetic maculopathy. *Invest Ophthalmol Vis Sci.* 2000; 41(1): 274–81.

56. Agardh E, Stjernquist H, Heijl A, Bengtsson B. Visual acuity and perimetry as measures of visual function in diabetic macular oedema. *Diabetologia.* 2006; 49(1): 200–6.

57. Bengtsson B, Heijl A, Agardh E. Visual fields correlate better than visual acuity to severity of diabetic retinopathy. *Diabetologia.* 2005; 48(12): 2494–500.

58. Heijl A, Lindgren G, Olsson HJ. A package for the statistical analysis of computerized visual fields. In: Greve EL, Heijl A, editors. *Seventh Internationl Visual Field Symposium.* Dordrecht, Boston, Lancaster: Martinus Nijhoff/Dr W. Junk Publishers; 1987; 153-68.

59. Bengtsson B, Lindgren A, Heijl A, Lindgren G, Asman P, Patella M. Perimetric probability maps to separate change caused by glaucoma from that caused by cataract. *Acta Ophthalmol Scand.* 1997; 75(2): 184–8.

60. Bengtsson B, Heijl A. A visual field index for calculation of glaucoma rate of progression. *Am J Ophthalmol.* 2008; 145(2): 343–53.

61. Andersson S, Heijl A, Bizios D, Bengtsson B. Comparison of clinicians and an artificial neural network regarding accuracy and certainty in performance of visual field assessment for the diagnosis of glaucoma. *Acta Ophthalmol.* 2012.

62. Åsman P, Heijl A. Evaluation of methods for automated Hemifield analysis in perimetry. *Arch Ophthalmol.* 1992; 110(6): 820–6.

63. Åsman P, Heijl A. Glaucoma Hemifield Test. Automated visual field evaluation. *Arch Ophthalmol.* 1992; 110(6): 812–9.

64. Katz J, Sommer A, Gaasterland DE, Anderson DR. Comparison of analytic algorithms for detecting glaucomatous visual field loss. *Arch Ophthalmol.* 1991; 109(12): 1684–9.

65. Heijl A LG, Olsson J. Reliability parameters in computerized perimetry. In: Greve EL, Heijl A, editors. *Seventh Internationl Visual Field Symposium.* Dordrecht, Boston, Lancaster: Martinus Nijhoff/Dr W. Junk Publishers; 1987; 593–600.

66. Katz J, Sommer A. Reliability indexes of automated perimetric tests. *Arch Ophthalmol.* 1988; 106(9): 1252–4.

67. Katz J, Sommer A. Reliability of automated perimetric tests. *Arch Ophthalmol.* 1990; 108(6): 777–8.

68. Katz J, Sommer A, Witt K. Reliability of visual field results over repeated testing. *Ophthalmology.* 1991; 98(1): 70–5.

69. Bengtsson B, Heijl A. False-negative responses in glaucoma perimetry: indicators of patient performance or test reliability? *Invest Ophthalmol Vis Sci.* 2000; 41(8): 2201–4.

70. Patella VM. How to Ascertain Progression and Outcome. In: Anderson DR, Drance SM, editors. *Encounters in Glaucoma Research 3.* Amsterdam: Kugler Publications; 1996. 183-93.

71. European Glaucoma Society. *Terminology and Guidelines for Glaucoma.* 3rd ed. Savona: Editrice Dogma S.r.l.; 2008.

72. Viswanathan AC, Crabb DP, McNaught AI, Westcott MC, Kamal D, Garway-Heath DF, et al. Interobserver agreement on visual field progression in glaucoma: a comparison of methods. *Br J Ophthalmol.* 2003; 87(6): 726–30.

73. Leske MC, Heijl A, Hyman L, Bengtsson B. Early Manifest Glaucoma Trial: design and baseline data. *Ophthalmology.* 1999; 106(11): 2144–53.

74. Tanna AP, Budenz DL, Bandi J, Feuer WJ, Feldman RM, Herndon LW, et al. Glaucoma Progression Analysis software compared with expert consensus opinion in the detection of visual field progression in glaucoma. *Ophthalmology.* 2012; 119(3): 468–73.

75. Artes PH, Chauhan BC, Keltner JL, Cello KE, Johnson CA, Anderson DR, et al. Longitudinal and cross-sectional analyses of visual field progression in participants of the Ocular Hypertension Treatment Study. *Arch Ophthalmol.* 2010; 128(12): 1528–32.

76. *Humphrey Field Analyzer User Manual.* Dublin, CA: Carl Zeiss Meditec, Inc.; 2010.

77. Heijl A LG, Lindgren A, Olsson J, Åsman P, Myers S, Patella VM. Extended empirical statistical package for evaluation of single and multiple fields in glaucoma: Statpac 2. In: Mills R, Heijl, A, editors. *Perimetry Update 1990-91.* Amsterdam, New York: Kulger Publications; 1991; 303-15.

78. Lee AC, Sample PA, Blumenthal EZ, Berry C, Zangwill L, Weinreb RN. Infrequent confirmation of visual field progression. *Ophthalmology.* 2002; 109(6): 1059–65.

79. Bengtsson B, Patella VM, Heijl A. Prediction of glaucomatous visual field loss by extrapolation of linear trends. *Arch Ophthalmol.* 2009; 127(12): 1610–5.

80. Koucheki B, Nouri-Mahdavi K, Patel G, Gaasterland D, Caprioli J. Visual field changes after cataract extraction: the AGIS experience. *Am J Ophthalmol.* 2004; 138(6): 1022–8.

81. Rao HL, Jonnadula GB, Addepalli UK, Senthil S, Garudadri CS. Effect of Cataract Extraction on Visual Field Index in Glaucoma. *J Glaucoma.* 2011.

82. Wall M, Johnson CA, Kutzko KE, Nguyen R, Brito C, Keltner JL. Long- and short-term variability of automated perimetry results in patients with optic neuritis and healthy subjects. *Arch Ophthalmol.* 1998; 116(1): 53–61.

83. Heijl A, Bengtsson, B. Early visual field defects in glaucoma: a study of eyes developing field loss. In: Bucci MG, editor. *Glaucoma: Decision Making in Therapy.* Milan: Springer-Verlag; 1996; 75-8.

84. Keltner JL, Johnson CA, Levine RA, Fan J, Cello KE, Kass MA, et al. Normal visual field test results following glaucomatous visual field end points in the Ocular Hypertension Treatment Study. *Arch Ophthalmol.* 2005; 123(9): 1201–6.

85. American Academy of Ophthalmology Glaucoma Panel. Preferred Practice Pattern Guidelines. Primary Open-Angle Glaucoma. San Francisco: American Academy of Ophthalmology; 2010.

86. Hyman LG, Komaroff E, Heijl A, Bengtsson B, Leske MC. Treatment and vision-related quality of life in the early manifest glaucoma trial. *Ophthalmology.* 2005; 112(9): 1505–13.

87. Turano KA, Rubin GS, Quigley HA. Mobility performance in glaucoma. *Invest Ophthalmol Vis Sci.* 1999; 40(12): 2803–9.

88. Jampel HD, Friedman DS, Quigley H, Miller R. Correlation of the binocular visual field with patient assessment of vision. *Invest Ophthalmol Vis Sci.* 2002; 43(4): 1059–67.

89. Jampel HD, Schwartz A, Pollack I, Abrams D, Weiss H, Miller R. Glaucoma patients' assessment of their visual function and quality of life. *J Glaucoma.* 2002; 11(2): 154–63.

90. McKean-Cowdin R, Wang Y, Wu J, Azen SP, Varma R. Impact of visual field loss on health-related quality of life in glaucoma: the Los Angeles Latino Eye Study. *Ophthalmology.* 2008; 115(6): 941–8 e1.

91. McKean-Cowdin R, Varma R, Wu J, Hays RD, Azen SP. Severity of visual field loss and health-related quality of life. *Am J Ophthalmol.* 2007; 143(6): 1013–23.

92. Friedman DS, Freeman E, Munoz B, Jampel HD, West SK. Glaucoma and mobility performance: the Salisbury Eye Evaluation Project. *Ophthalmology.* 2007; 114(12): 2232–7.

93. Glen FC, Crabb DP, Smith ND, Burton R, Garway-Heath DF. Do patients with glaucoma have difficulty recognizing faces? *Invest Ophthalmol Vis Sci.* 2012; 53(7): 3629–37.

94. Ramulu PY, van Landingham SW, Massof RW, Chan ES, Ferrucci L, Friedman DS. Fear of falling and visual field loss from glaucoma. *Ophthalmology.* 2012; 119(7): 1352–8.

95. Saunders LJ, Russell RA, Crabb DP. Practical landmarks for visual field disability in glaucoma. *Br J Ophthalmol.* 2012.

96. Jampel HD, Vitale S, Ding Y, Quigley H, Friedman D, Congdon N, et al. Test-retest variability in structural and functional parameters of glaucoma damage in the glaucoma imaging longitudinal study. *J Glaucoma.* 2006; 15(2): 152–7.

97. Chauhan BC, Garway-Heath DF, Goni FJ, Rossetti L, Bengtsson B, Viswanathan AC, et al. Practical recommendations for measuring rates of visual field change in glaucoma. *Br J Ophthalmol.* 2008; 92(4): 569–73.

98. Stein JD, Talwar N, Laverne AM, Nan B, Lichter PR. Trends in use of ancillary glaucoma tests for patients with open-angle glaucoma from 2001 to 2009. *Ophthalmology.* 2012; 119(4): 748–58.

99. Grødum K, Heijl A, Bengtsson B. A comparison of glaucoma patients identified through mass screening and in routine clinical practice. *Acta Ophthalmol Scand.* 2002; 80(6): 627–31.

100. Kass MA, Heuer DK, Higginbotham EJ, Johnson CA, Keltner JL, Miller JP, et al. The Ocular Hypertension Treatment Study: a randomized trial determines that topical ocular hypotensive medication delays or prevents the onset of primary open-angle glaucoma. *Arch Ophthalmol.* 2002; 120(6): 701–13; discussion 829–30.

101. Burr J, Botello-Pinzon P, Takwoingi Y, Hernandez R, Vazquez-Montes M, Elders A, et al. Surveillance for ocular hypertension: an evidence synthesis and economic evaluation. *Health Technol Assess.* 2012; 16(29): 1–272.

102. Leske MC, Heijl A, Hyman L, Bengtsson B, Dong L, Yang Z. Predictors of long-term progression in the early manifest glaucoma trial. *Ophthalmology.* 2007; 114(11): 1965–72.

103. Heijl A, Lindgren G, Olsson J. The effect of perimetric experience in normal subjects. *Arch Ophthalmol.* 1989; 107(1): 81–6.

104. Wild JM, Searle AE, Dengler-Harles M, O'Neill EC. Long-term follow-up of baseline learning and fatigue effects in the automated perimetry of glaucoma and ocular hypertensive patients. *Acta Ophthalmol.* 1991; 69(2): 210–6.

105. Heijl A, Bengtsson B. The effect of perimetric experience in patients with glaucoma. *Arch Ophthalmol.* 1996; 114(1): 19–22.

106. Gardiner SK, Demirel S, Johnson CA. Is there evidence for continued learning over multiple years in perimetry? *Optom Vis Sci.* 2008; 85(11): 1043–8.

107. Anderson DR, Drance SM, Schulzer M. Natural history of normal-tension glaucoma. *Ophthalmology.* 2001; 108(2): 247–53.

108. Heijl A, Bengtsson B, Hyman L, Leske MC. Natural history of open-angle glaucoma. *Ophthalmology.* 2009; 116(12): 2271–6.

109. Ahrlich KG, De Moraes CG, Teng CC, Prata TS, Tello C, Ritch R, et al. Visual field progression differences between normal-tension and exfoliative high-tension glaucoma. *Invest Ophthalmol Vis Sci.* 2010; 51(3): 1458–63.

110. Heijl A BP, Norrgren G, Bengtsson B. Rates of visual field progression in clinical glaucoma care. *Acta Ophthalmol,* accepted for publicatiom. 2012.

111. Heijl A, Leske MC, Bengtsson B, Hyman L, Hussein M. Reduction of intraocular pressure and glaucoma progression: results from the Early Manifest Glaucoma Trial. *Arch Ophthalmol.* 2002; 120(10): 1268–79.

112. Folgar FA, De Moraes CG, Teng CC, Tello C, Ritch R, Liebmann JM. Effect of Successful and Partly Successful Filtering Surgery on the Velocity of Glaucomatous Visual Field Progression. *J Glaucoma.* 2011.

113. De Moraes CG, Demirel S, Gardiner SK, Liebmann JM, Cioffi GA, Ritch R, et al. Effect of treatment on the rate of visual field change in the ocular hypertension treatment study observation group. *Invest Ophthalmol Vis Sci.* 2012; 53(4): 1704–9.

114. Weinreb RN, Garway-Heath DF, Leung C, Crowston JG, Medeiros FA. *Progression of Glaucoma.* The Hague: Kugler Publications; 2011.

115. Crabb DP, Garway-Heath DF. Intervals between visual field tests when monitoring the glaucomatous patient: wait-and-see approach. *Invest Ophthalmol Vis Sci.* 2012; 53(6): 2770–6.

116. Nouri-Mahdavi K, Zarei R, Caprioli J. Influence of visual field testing frequency on detection of glaucoma progression with trend analyses. *Arch Ophthalmol.* 2011; 129(12): 1521–7.

117. Iester M, Mikelberg FS, Courtright P, Drance SM. Correlation between the visual field indices and Heidelberg retina tomograph parameters. *J Glaucoma.* 1997; 6(2): 78–82.

118. Chauhan BC, McCormick TA, Nicolela MT, LeBlanc RP. Optic disc and visual field changes in a prospective longitudinal study of patients with glaucoma: comparison of scanning laser tomography with conventional perimetry and optic disc photography. *Arch Ophthalmol.* 2001; 119(10): 1492–9.

119. Artes PH, Chauhan BC. Longitudinal changes in the visual field and optic disc in glaucoma. *Prog Retin Eye Res.* 2005; 24(3): 333–54.

120. Hood DC, Anderson SC, Wall M, Raza AS, Kardon RH. A test of a linear model of glaucomatous structure-function loss reveals sources of variability in retinal nerve fiber and visual field measurements. *Invest Ophthalmol Vis Sci.* 2009; 50(9): 4254–66.

121. Zhu H, Crabb DP, Fredette MJ, Anderson DR, Garway-Heath DF. Quantifying discordance between structure and function measurements in the clinical assessment of glaucoma. *Arch Ophthalmol.* 2011; 129(9): 1167–74.

122. Leite MT, Zangwill LM, Weinreb RN, Rao HL, Alencar LM, Medeiros FA. Structure-function relationships using the Cirrus spectral domain optical coherence tomograph and standard automated perimetry. *J Glaucoma.* 2012; 21(1): 49–54.

123. Keltner JL, Johnson CA, Anderson DR, Levine RA, Fan J, Cello KE, et al. The association between glaucomatous visual fields and optic nerve head features in the Ocular Hypertension Treatment Study. *Ophthalmology.* 2006; 113(9): 1603–12.

124. Kerrigan-Baumrind LA, Quigley HA, Pease ME, Kerrigan DF, Mitchell RS. Number of ganglion cells in glaucoma eyes compared with threshold visual field tests in the same persons. *Invest Ophthalmol Vis Sci.* 2000; 41(3): 741–8.

125. Bizios D, Heijl A, Bengtsson B. Integration and fusion of standard automated perimetry and optical coherence tomography data for improved automated glaucoma diagnostics. *BMC Ophthalmol.* 2011; 11: 20.

126. Medeiros FA, Zangwill LM, Girkin CA, Liebmann JM, Weinreb RN. Combining structural and functional measurements to improve estimates of rates of glaucomatous progression. *Am J Ophthalmol.* 2012; 153(6): 1197–205 e1.

127. Russell RA, Malik R, Chauhan BC, Crabb DP, Garway-Heath DF. Improved estimates of visual field progression using bayesian linear regression to integrate structural information in patients with ocular hypertension. *Invest Ophthalmol Vis Sci.* 2012; 53(6): 2760–9.

128. Nevalainen J, Krapp E, Paetzold J, Mildenberger I, Besch D, Vonthein R, et al. Visual field defects in acute optic neuritis--distribution of different types of defect pattern, assessed with threshold-related supraliminal perimetry, ensuring high spatial resolution. *Graefes Arch Clin Exp Ophthalmol.* 2008; 246(4): 599–607.

129. Keltner JL, Johnson CA, Cello KE, Dontchev M, Gal RL, Beck RW. Visual field profile of optic neuritis: a final follow-up report from the optic neuritis treatment trial from baseline through 15 years. *Arch Ophthalmol.* 2010; 128(3): 330–7.

130. Trick GL, Trick LR, Kilo C. Visual field defects in patients with insulin-dependent and noninsulin-dependent diabetes. *Ophthalmology.* 1990; 97(4): 475–82.

131. Henricsson M, Heijl A. Visual fields at different stages of diabetic retinopathy. *Acta Ophthalmol* (Copenh). 1994; 72(5): 560–9.

132. Wild JM, Dengler-Harles M, Searle AE, O'Neill EC, Crews SJ. The influence of the learning effect on automated perimetry in patients with suspected glaucoma. *Acta Ophthalmol.* 1989; 67(5): 537–45.

133. Johnson CA, Cioffi GA, Drance SM, Gaasterland D, Mills RP, Ashburn F, et al. A multicenter comparison study of the Humphrey Field Analyzer I and the Humphrey Field Analyzer II. *Ophthalmology.* 1997; 104(11): 1910–7.

134. Andersson S, Heijl A, Boehm AG, Bengtsson B. The effect of education on the assessment of optic nerve head photographs for the glaucoma diagnosis. *BMC Ophthalmol.* 2011; 11: 12.

Index

Swedish Interactive Thresholding Algorithm Standard. *See* SITA Standard

T

technician. *See* perimetrist
temporal raphe, 79
10-2 pattern, 4, 30, 32, 34-37, 45
test-retest variability, 2, 66
30-2 fields, 9, 29, 30, 32, 34-37, 45, 135, 136
threshold sensitivity, 6, 24, 47, 54
threshold testing, 3, 27
thyroid ophthalmopathy, 118-119
total deviation, 47, 49
Total Deviation decibel map, 47
Total Deviation probability plots, 4, 47, 53
trial lens artifacts, 135-136
trial lenses, 13-14
"trigger-happy" patients, 9, 49, 52, 138, 139
tumors, 76-78
24-2 fields, 9, 27, 29, 32, 34-37, 45, 132, 135

U

U.S. Social Security Administration, disability determinations, 33

V

VFI. *See* Visual Field Index
visual field
  normal, 5, 21
  sensitivity, 25, 26
Visual Field Index (VFI), 6, 7, 53, 68, 69-70, 71, 72-74, 98-100
visual field loss
  artifactual field loss, 6, 49, 131-142
  congruity, 124
  generalized, 84
  in glaucoma, 2, 79-87, 89, 97
  homogeneous, 84
  in lesions of optic chiasm, 120-121
  localized, 22, 84
  in neurological disease, 2, 111-124

in optic nerve disease, 111-119
in postchiasmal lesions, 122-123
quality of life (QOL) and, 89
in retinal disease, 2, 125-129
test-retest variability, 2, 66
types, 22, 84
visual field progression
  in glaucoma, 6, 61-71, 94, 96
  in other diseases, 71
visual field sensitivity, 25, 26
visual field testing
  artifactual loss, 6, 131-142
  baseline tests, 94
  "filling-in" effect, 22, 23
  in glaucoma, 1, 4, 6, 7, 30, 32, 34-37
  interpretation pitfalls, 9
  in neurological disease, 1, 30
  nonspecific findings, 22
  in other diseases, 76-77
  in retinal disease, 2, 30
  testing frequency, 97
  See also perimetry